The
Put Your Money
Where Your Mouth Is
Diet Book

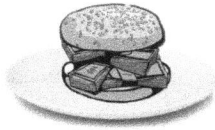

The Ultimate Companion
for Unstoppable Weight Loss

Daniel R. Miller

Put Your Money Where Your Mouth Is:
The Ultimate Companion for Unstoppable Weight Loss
by Daniel R. Miller

Published by Lifestyle Services

Book design: Nick Zelinger, www.NZGraphics.com

ISBN: 978-0-615-98316-5

First Edition

Printed in the United States of America

This book is dedicated to my
little brother Michael Nahum Miller
whose eternal presence in my life is a gift
in more ways than words can ever describe.

CONTENTS

Foreword

It could have just as easily been called Walking Your Talk, Standing in Your Own Truth, Living with Integrity—any number of little sayings that capture the essence of making a commitment, most importantly, to *yourself*.

Daniel R. Miller's new book, *Put Your Money Where Your Mouth Is*, takes a light-hearted and whimsical approach to the emotionally-charged, and "heavy," subject of weight loss. Obesity has become epidemic, faddish diets rise and fall faster and with the same predictability as the tides, and information taken as absolute and indisputable truth today is disproved, dismissed and replaced tomorrow.

What's the answer? According to MIller, whose body morphed during the process of writing his book into a strong and fit physique, while his spirit soared with self-confidence, it doesn't really matter what diet you're on. Yes, there are prescriptive measures a person might have to take for this or that set of conditions, but even so, without the "missing ingredient" failure to sustain the discipline or regimen required is almost preordained—even if it's a matter of life or death.

The missing ingredient is commitment, self-accountability. It wasn't easy for Daniel to lose the 80 pounds he had to shed to get down to his goal of 180 pounds; he admits that writing the book was fraught with challenges and frustrations to the point of just wanting to throw in the towel. But he didn't, he stuck it out to completion, and now can enjoy the accomplishment of being 80 pounds lighter and a published author.

Daniel has accomplished many things on his personal journey. The school of life has taught him many no nonsense principles. He is a man of conviction. When he sees a part he can play to help the world, he learns that part and plays it well. I admire the way he has used his education and sought opportunities to excel in all that he set out to accomplish. That's walking the talk, standing in one's truth, living with integrity.

Put Your Money Where Your Mouth Is is a unique self-help book. The author is a free spirit (he has an Apache father) with an adventurous character. Recently we spent a full day together discussing his business model, branding and marketing strategy, product development, potential profit centers and the like. Before beginning we went outside to offer a prayer to the "Big Spirit" just in time to observe a red tale hawk journey by to give us its blessings. Oho!

Daniel's intense level of personal commitment and persistence will carry the day. He's inspiring and will succeed, and in the process he will help thousands of people understand that diet is more about what's goes in between your ears than in your mouth.

Oho, brother, oho!

James Alvino, Ph.D
Business and Success Coach

Chapter 1

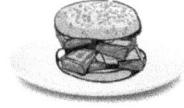

Why I Want You To Succeed

I know yo-yo dieting. I have gained and lost the same 25 pounds more times than I care to remember.

After creating my own Mexican restaurant, my own tequila bar, and my own construction business, I found that I had also created a pear-shaped body that I could not get rid of with my own willpower. Being an overachiever, I found this extremely frustrating.

Then, just by luck, I happened upon a demonstration that changed my life. I learned the secret to losing weight and keeping it off. Hint: It is not a nutritional secret.

I love food. I love alcohol. I love partying. I love life. I love creating new ideas that make other people happy. Unfortunately, I also have an addictive personality. I gain weight just by looking at yummy foods. My resistance is low. My appetites are high. Can you relate?

Let's back up to where my problem started. When my kids were young, I started a Mexican Taqueria in Olympia, Washington. The Mexican food in that town was pretty "saucy" when I got there so I felt inspired to do something about it. Burrito Heaven was a line-out-the-door establishment that served "burritos the size of your forearm," as the local newspaper put it.

To make matters even more fun, I started The Tequila Bar. We featured 100% agave tequila. We even gave out bachelor's degrees in "tequiliology", if you sampled enough of our products.

So I got paid to eat and drink and hang out and chat and have fun and get fat. I didn't have a lot of time to go running.

After our second child, Rylie, was born, my then-wife and I sold the bar and the restaurant and moved to the country to raise our kids amid nature spirits instead of alcohol spirits. I bought a backhoe and became a heavy equipment operator. In a matter of 30 days my employee situation transformed from over forty employees to just one… me. I was still sitting around; only now it was on the seat of the tractor instead of a bar stool.

My gut hung over my belt. It jiggled and vibrated to the tone of the diesel engine. My tractor carried my extra weight happily, but my back and knees did not. I knew I had to do something about all the extra fat I had put on. I found it difficult to stay committed to a diet, when I had so many other commitments to attend to: my wife and kids, my new job, and our new home. My family and I didn't merely buy a new home in the country; we built it ourselves. We put in solar and water power. We built a wonderful pond for swimming and fishing.

Kathleen shared in all of it. Plus, she was the one who had gone through carrying both our children for nine months each. She didn't have the weight problem I did. She had long since shed her baby weight, and she looked beautiful. Yet, no matter how inspired I was, both by her and my own desire to be my best, I still struggled with those extra 25 pounds.

When heavy equipment operation turned into real estate investing, Kathleen and I took some classes. Surprisingly, at one of these classes I came across the creative idea that would unlock my secret for losing the pounds I so wanted to get rid of. It started with a key word: Commitment. Commitment alone wasn't enough. This commitment had to come from outside myself.

In real estate investing, I found that I was not as motivated to perform when I had something to gain as I was when I had something to lose. So I decided to apply this realization in my approach to weight loss.

I care about people, so I want to share this with you.

If you're reading this book, then you have most likely tried and failed at other weight loss programs. I understand that. I did too. I would hear about a diet, try it, lose a few pounds, and get all excited and tell my friends about it. Then something would inevitably send me off course: a celebration, a bachelor party, a vacation, a night out… You know what I mean. I would cheat and fall off my diet. I told myself it was just for one night. I would feel bloated and ashamed. I would eat and drink my way deeper into my shame, until my diet became a distant dark hole somewhere in the recesses of my brain.

I want to applaud you for giving it one more shot by reading this book. I have found the method I'm about to share to truly be the missing link for me. I believe it may well be the missing link for you, too.

I believe that where you are right now is exactly where you are supposed to be. Love yourself for where you are. Forgive yourself for your mistakes and failures.

Nothing in life happens in a straight line. Life is a series of peaks and valleys, and I believe it's up to us to find joy in all of them. Look at any graph of any successful stock, and if you look closely you'll see many ups and downs. In time, the line still moves upward. Maybe you're in a valley right now. I sincerely hope this book will take you to a peak. I hope my personally tested ideas will help you commit to the body of your dreams.

Although my method bypasses the usual approaches to weight loss, commitment is still key. Your health is far more important than anything else in your life. Without it, the rest doesn't matter. If you don't see it that way and are not willing to make your health as important as your rent or your mortgage, then I suggest you stop reading this book right now.

Are you still with me? Good. I can assure you that nothing tastes better than being slender feels.

The techniques suggested in this book are all backed up by modern psychology and neuroscience. Much of what brain researchers have discovered tells me that we have been focusing on the wrong motivations in our fight against obesity. With the systems enclosed in this book you can change weight loss from a grueling, losing battle into a fun, adventurous, humorous journey.

Put Your Money Where Your Mouth Is is not meant to be a stand-alone diet book, but a companion book that will help you succeed at whatever healthy diet you do choose. That means these techniques work well with any and all healthy diets or weight loss programs. Although I'm a certified nutritionist, I do not deal with any nutritional matters in this book. I'm also a holistic health practitioner and hypnotherapist, but I won't be talking about that either. In all of my studies of nutrition, the main thing I've learned is that there is no one way to get there; so I stay out of it. I know what nutritional programs work for me, but I don't claim to know what diets work for you.

Although I won't steer you toward any particular diet, I do have confidence in the power of solid contracts and agreements. I have a good understanding of what motivates and inspires people. Perhaps the most important thing my technique does is to help you stay focused on your goal through the inevitable dips in the process. Better than that, this technique actually carries you through the difficult times when "willpower" cannot.

This technique is going to use of the network of people in your life to create a support team unlike any support system you've leaned on before. The more experience I have, the more I know that I need other people to help me accomplish big things in life. Believe me; overcoming the emotional and physical barriers to transforming your body is one of the biggest things one can accomplish in life.

Although the diet you pick is up to you, I do recommend that you see a physician before beginning any weight loss program. This book focuses primarily on helping you stick to your commitment when the going gets tough.

Welcome to my program! I want to assure you that all my suggestions are safe. They're powerful as well. If you commit to this program, you will definitely see results. As with anything in life, if you are not getting the results you want, you probably just need to add more commitment. I'm here to show you how to do just that.

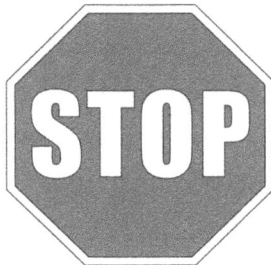

Stop

Now how many books do you know that start with a stop sign? This is not some liability warning, but an honest-to-God "Stop!"

I believe all of us are connected, so I really care about all people, wherever we may meet, even in the pages of a book. That means I truly care about you and your success. I care about you feeling good in your body, feeling good in your clothes, feeling good about being the person you are on this planet…

Because I care about you, I want to know whether you are really serious about losing the weight you say you want to lose. If you're not really serious, then please put down this book or pass it on to a friend. Here's why: Every time you go on a diet and fail, your self-esteem takes a hit. The process of dieting and failing is one of the biggest causes of obesity in America today. If you are not absolutely certain that you are willing to do what it takes to lose your excess fat, then you will fail. When we fail, sometimes we feel ashamed. When we feel ashamed, sometimes we overeat. I don't want you to fail.

My mission is to help end obesity in the world. If my book serves to make people fatter, as many diet books do, then I am working against myself. So please decide whether you are committed to doing what it takes to lose weight.

If you're not committed, please do us both a favor: Don't contribute to me failing at my mission. Stop reading now.

If you are committed to doing what it takes to lose your excess weight, read on. Think of me as a guide; someone who will lead you through the process of getting to the body you want. If you get thinner, more self-confident, cuter, happier, buy better-fitting clothes, become more attractive to your mate, or get the mate of your dreams, then your happiness makes the world a happier place. People will notice when you lose weight. They'll be impressed because they themselves have tried to lose weight. Whether they succeeded or failed, they know it is an undertaking that requires commitment.

Do you ever feel alone in your relationship with food? That's right, it is a relationship. It is personal. It's your responsibility, but you are not alone. According to the Food Research and Action Center, 68% of Americans are either overweight or obese. When you're overweight it pervades your life on all levels: body, mind, and spirit. Carrying excess fat taxes your body and can contribute to many diseases, such as diabetes and heart disease. It's tough on your mind because it can cause shame, lack of self-confidence, and increased experiences of unfair discrimination in society. It's hard on your spirit because it saps your energy and capacity for joy during your limited time on this planet.

I have felt alone in my struggle with weight. I often dieted while raising two kids who did not, so I made separate dishes most of the time. I still ate "little tastes" of the "kid food" that was around. It tasted so good and felt so nurturing… for a moment; but it was so non-nutritional that sometimes I can't even believe I fed that junk to my boys.

In an effort to avoid gaining weight from all my cheating, I was up early exercising every morning before driving my kids to the bus stop for school. Sometimes I resented the fact that my kids could eat as much as they wanted and not get fat, and that my friends seemed to be able to eat as much as they wanted and not get fat.

Why was I the only one I knew who was obsessed by my excess weight? How could something as simple as 25 pounds of fat defeat me?

The Difficulty with Commitment

What is commitment? We think we know. We're asked for it all the time. Although we might not think about it, we make a commitment every time we go to the grocery store and trade our money for food and drink. What are we committing to? Survival? Health? Enjoyment? A lifestyle?

What are we committed to in life? Our next breath of air? The well-being of our families, friends, and pets? Clean water and healthy food? Making a home? Maybe we're committed to something beyond the basics: financial success, saving the environment, having fun, social justice, creating art, playing music…

A man on the streets of New York is asking directions, "Do you know the way to Carnegie Hall?" A helpful citizen answers, "Practice, practice, practice." That old joke might be funny, but it's also true. If you want to make great music, it's all about commitment. If you want to get your body in shape, that's all about commitment, too.

If your body is not fit, it's not your fault. You just were not committed to the level necessary to make that kind of change in your body. Maybe you didn't realize how much commitment it would take. Or maybe you did, and you thought that much commitment would be too hard. That's not true. *The commitment makes it easier, not harder.*

Most diets have a motivational component,
but lack a true commitment component.

Commitment is a two-way street. A commitment is between two people. Eating is a one-way street. The food goes in one way and comes out the other. How do we go about converting a one way process to a two-way commitment? First, allow me to explain why the commitments you made before didn't work.

Evolution works against you. Your primal reptilian brain works against you. Your primal reptilian brain is a force to be reckoned with in your decision-making process. It loves to hoard and store. It hates change. It hates to step outside its comfort zone. Your reptilian brain is the one that you watch working the refrigerator for seconds and thirds even though you know it's unhealthy. It's the out-of-control beast that diminishes your self-esteem. When you want to lose weight, it's the primitive part of your brain that stacks the neurological and psychological odds against you.

Motivation Is Not the Same as Commitment

All the positive motivation and self-talk in the world will not convince the reptilian brain that it should stop hoarding energy. That typically means eating as much as possible and exercising as little as necessary. So if you want to lose weight, you have to convince the entire nervous system that it's beneficial to give up stored energy and get fit. I have created a system that helps you do that by aligning all the energies of your being: mind, body, and spirit. No woo-woo metaphysics. Just basic stuff.

This is not a nutritional diet program. After having studied many different philosophies on nutrition, I have concluded that the jury is still out. Some things work for some people, some things work for other people, but commitment works for everybody. This is a diet "companion" book that will supercharge whatever nutrition-based diet you choose.

Whether we eat nutritious food or junk food, we all like to eat. We like yummy food that tastes good in our mouths and feels good in our bellies. It puts us in our comfort zone. I bring this up because if you commit to losing weight, it's going to take you out of your comfort zone. I'll do my best to make this easy and fun, but it won't be comfortable. Don't worry. As you may have already discovered, life is more fun outside the comfort zone anyway.

Making a commitment does not guarantee that you will make progress every step of the way.

If you charted anybody's progress in transforming their body, you would see that the graph always moves up and down along the path to success. This is also true of people who overcome serious illness, except that on their "down" days they may come close to death. Although your weight issue might not be quite that dire, don't underestimate the comparison. If you're obese, sooner or later it could be a life or death situation. Even if you're merely overweight, then losing the excess weight is still a physical recovery situation. This is not kids stuff, whether you need to lose 25 pounds or 200 pounds.

You will not only face up and down days on your way to losing weight. You will also experience up and down days in your recovery from the physical and emotional damage you endured when you were out of shape.

Motivation is something you will feel on your up days. But your commitment to get through this no matter what is what will get you through your down days.

Personally, I have failed so many times that it almost felt like a habit. But all those past failures only make me that much more grateful today at having found my way through.

I have discovered there is only one reason why people fail to lose weight. They fail because they don't understand how to make a commitment at the level required to succeed.

Deep commitment always finds a way to success. It's just a matter of knowing how to make the kind of commitment that sticks.

Deep commitment claws and hacks its way to success. Deep commitment keeps asking questions and investigating. It does not give up until it finds an answer. Deep commitment has hope, optimism, and confidence in a successful outcome. I'm positive there is already something in your own life, no matter who you are, that you are committed to at that level. Whatever it is in your life that you committed to so completely that you would never entertain the alternative, that is the level of commitment

19

you need if you're going to succeed at achieving personal health. Anything less works against you. Anything less makes it almost impossible to succeed. It's a big deal to change the shape of your body. So treat it like a big deal.

Of Course it's Hard

Do you love to lose weight, but hate dieting? Of course you do. I believe that's primarily because the term "diet" has been perverted until it no longer bears a relationship to its original meaning: "what a person or animal eats." The term diet no longer seems to bear any relationship to normal living. Instead, it's associated with the ideas of deprivation and failure. Some people try to distance themselves from the stigma of such words as diet and exercise by renaming them things such as a cleanse, a detox, a fitness program, a purge, etc...

It doesn't matter what word you use for your approach to transforming your body. If you don't make an unbreakable commitment, you probably won't succeed.

When I ask you to make a commitment to your goal, I won't tell you what kind of goal to set. You can measure success in pounds, kilos, inches, centimeters, body fat ratio, or clothing size. I think it would be fun to figure out a way to define success in terms of a six-pack. The nice thing about all of the above examples is that they are measurable. You cannot cheat a number.

So long as you're prepared to commit to some sort of measurable number, I guarantee this book will give you success on whatever diet you choose. I can help you make some decisions about dieting, but I will not promote or criticize any particular diet. You supply the diet and I'll supply the commitment.

I will tell you that whatever dietary approach you choose, I have probably done some version of it. I've lost weight on a lot of different diets. I always gained it back when I started cheating. I couldn't recover from my cheating because I hadn't figured out how to make an *unbreakable commitment*. For me the diet always ended when I stopped regularly weighing myself on my scale.

When I finally had long-lasting success at controlling my weight, people started asking me what kind of exercise I do. I tell them it doesn't matter what kind of exercise I do, because they need to do what works for them. Whatever type of diet or exercise program you choose, just remember what my dad taught me: It's easier if you make it an adventure, see it as a game, or make a challenge of it. Take every opportunity to laugh and smile. When you make a mistake, laugh at that too. Whatever you do, make sure it's something you enjoy so that you will stay motivated. It's the person you will become when the diet is done that you need to fall in love with now.

Chapter 2

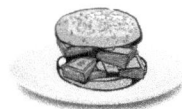

An Unbreakable Commitment

Although I'm a certified nutritionist, as well as a body worker, holistic healer, and polarity therapist, I don't claim to know enough about diet, nutrition, or health to be an authority. I'll leave it to people with fancy letters after their names to guide you in that arena. I'd prefer you to think of me as just a normal guy who has dealt with both food and alcohol addiction, made a lot of mistakes trying to overcome both, yet has finally found a path to long-term success. I've discovered how to make the kind of commitment to my body that now allows me to live a joyful, healthy life with my kids.

I admit: I still love fat. I love bacon, sausage, salsa, Zen pancakes, ice cream, caramel, buttered popcorn, and Oreos. I love food and drink that overwhelms my senses. If I were to break my commitments, I could eat until I was so stuffed it hurt, and drink until I couldn't see straight.

I remember one binge when my kids were coming home for a visit; one from college, and one from boarding school. The day before they arrived, I went to the big grocery store in the big city nearby and got a good deal on lots of teen-style treats. I bought *Drumstick* ice cream cones and caramel-filled vanilla ice cream bars. I also bought some healthy *Weight Watchers* bars. I ate all the *Weight Watchers* bars on the way home. That night, I ate the entire box of *Drumsticks* ice cream cones with the chocolate and nut coating, along with buttered popcorn. The next night, before my kids arrived, I felt compelled to return to the freezer for the ice-cream bars. I polished off that box and some more buttered popcorn while watching the World Series.

Even as I walked toward that freezer full of ice cream, I knew I could resist temptation for a while. I also knew in the back of my mind that temptation would win. So I rationalized, "Well, I can fight this urge for a couple of hours, but I'm going to lose anyway. So I might as well start eating them now." As for the popcorn, I popped some of the expensive stuff with essential fatty acids, and told myself that this would help me fight off Alzheimer's. I enjoyed my feast of sugar and fat thoroughly. Luckily, my sweet girlfriend brought some ice cream over so there would still be some by the time my boys arrived.

I realize that thinking was pretty screwed up. Perhaps the saddest part is that I had just finished a weight loss program that had taken my weight down to 175. I was looking good with my six-pack abs. I got there with a low carbohydrate, low lactose diet—which I do not endorse. The point is that I had barely tasted success before I stopped following the rules... rules I had set for myself. I was backsliding, big time.

I told you this story for two reasons:

1. So you know that I will be honest with you in this book.

2. So you understand that I am just a normal guy who has problems like you. I am not some scientist in a lab figuring out the best food combination to create the best hormonal balance to trick the body into dropping fat. That is not my domain.

Now let me tell you what my big mistake was. I only made a commitment to myself to maintain my goal-weight, and did not make a commitment to anyone else. I discovered the hard way that I don't accomplish nearly as much in my life unless I make appointments, arrangements, and commitments. I do best at keeping my commitments when I make them to other people, and when I commit to paying big consequences if I break those commitments.

Our primitive reptilian brain responds to commitments when it has something to lose.

I have seen my approach to commitment work first-hand. It's like getting into an elevator in a hotel tower and punching a button. You choose which floor you want to reach; you punch that number, and down you go. The scariest thing is pushing the button. Why? For me, it's because I put my money where my mouth is. When I make a commitment to lose or maintain my weight, I make that commitment to another person; and in case I fail to perform, I promise to pay a penalty so big it will hurt. That makes it scary, because I know that if I push that button that means I absolutely am going to change. There is no alternative. I have made an unbreakable commitment.

Once you make an unbreakable commitment, there's no question: you're going to face and overcome your subconscious motivations for overeating. The system I've created will help you do so as a natural part of the process. Not only will you be transforming your body, but you will also be entering a period of personal growth. You need to change your way of thinking about things, and making an unbreakable commitment is the first step towards doing that. Once you push that button, you are strapped in with no choice but to change. When you realize that, it will rock your world. You will feel lighter, even before you lose the first pound.

If I can help one person latch onto this commitment system and feel better in body and mind, as well as in relationship with the world and other people, then writing this book will be worth it. For me, this is a path to service, and service equals happiness.

Chapter 3

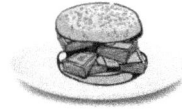

Everybody Cheats On Diets

R eally? Doesn't somebody, anybody, stick to a diet 100% of the time? I defy you to find that person. Go ahead. Ask around. But if someone tells you they never cheat, be suspicious. Be very suspicious.

When Do Diets Work?

Here's my definition of a diet: a list of items you put in your mouth, chew, and swallow. For most of us there is a pattern to that, though the pattern varies from person to person. Back in the hunter-gatherer days of our ancestors, humans mostly ate whatever the other people in their tribe ate, because that was all there was: game, plants, nuts and berries.

Today there are wines and cheeses, burgers and fries, canned veggies and fruit juices, ice cream and soda, and cookies, cakes and candies. These things can keep some of us going just great, until one day we hit a wall, maybe at age 30, 40, or 50. When some people start gaining weight they've never seen before, they panic and try extreme diets. Some of them work great for a while, until people get hungry or frustrated and give up. Then there is the "exercise like crazy and eat anything I want" diet. That works for some people too, until it doesn't. Many of us end up on this diet, then that diet, then the "I'll try anything" diet, then another. That was me.

Of course, sometimes doctors put us on diets to help treat serious diseases, such as diabetes, cancer, or heart disease. If you're on a doctor-recommended diet, make sure you still follow the rules for that diet when I ask you to make your new commitment.

It's tough to face the "D" word; but if you want to lose weight, you're definitely going to have to change your eating habits (which is another way of saying you have to change your diet). That's the only sure way to lose weight.

So if we want to lose weight, why do we think of the "D" word as such a bad word? Why do people associate "diet" with failure? I don't believe it's because everybody cheats. I believe it's because most people don't know how to get back on track *after* they cheat.

Let me tell you a way to make better use of your time when you do your informal survey in search of that one person who never cheated on a diet. Focus on those people who say they cheated on a diet, but who lost weight anyway and are still in great shape. Ask them, "How did you get back on track? How did you overcome your bad habits? How did you achieve your goal despite setbacks?"

I'm confident you'll find that the people who succeeded at losing weight, despite the urge to cheat, either created a high level of commitment to themselves, or they made some form of a commitment to someone aside from themselves.

Accepting the Roller Coaster

Most modern diet books suggest ways to allow "treats" into your weight loss formula. Many diets provide some sort of outlet for a sugar craving. Many diets have a means of counting calories so that we know when it's time to stop eating. But do any of those things put a lid on our urges? Does all our knowledge about what is healthy or unhealthy, fattening or non-fattening, stop us from going to the refrigerator, restaurant, or store and grabbing that favorite little snack that we know will taste so delicious on our tongue? What makes it harder is that we know that it will take hardly any effort to enjoy that snack right *now*, while it could take months of effort before our body looks the way we want it to.

Take a moment and consider all the ways you've cheated on diets. I know it's embarrassing. We're talking out-of-control behavior, ridiculous rationalizations, and pointless lies. But guess what? I'm not going to tell you how to shut off the urge to cheat. Instead, I'm going to help you get back on track before one little cheat turns into all-out diet anarchy.

No healing of any kind happens in a straight line of perfect progress. So the first thing you need to do is give up expecting that.

One of my best friends once landed in the hospital with severe burns over 70% of his body. For the first week, he did better than expected, talking, flirting with the nurses, and holding warm conversations with loved ones who came to visit. We were all amazed. Then his nurse took a few of us into another room and gave us the bad news.

"Your friend is in what we call a honeymoon period." she said. "Here in the burn unit we see it all the time. He may look good now, but there will be some ups and downs in his healing process." She took a black marker and drew a line on a whiteboard, a line with ups and downs just like a stock chart. She told us that this was what his progress would be like as he recovered.

What we didn't realize at the time was that those dips and troughs she drew would represent near-death experiences for my friend. During those times, his doctors and nurses were busy doing everything they could to resuscitate him, to kill deadly bacteria, and to keep his organs from failing. For three months on his path to recovery, he was in what I would now call a coma. He remembers nothing from that period. Miraculously, he survived and now leads forays into the jungles of Brazil.

That's when I got the concept on a deeper level; success truly does not happen in a straight line. Changing habits need not be a near-death experience, but it's still not easy. Everybody cheats on diets. The successful dieters are the ones who cheat and come out of it. They find a way to turn a trough into a peak. They find the strength to throw the cookies into the driveway for the birds or the dogs to eat. They make some kind of a statement or take some kind of action that tells the world that they are through with this addictive behavior.

So if you are overweight, and you have dieted and failed in the past, remember: you are just in a dip. You are not a failure, but a work-in-progress. If you have dieted and lost weight only to put it all back on, you have simply learned one of the many ways not to diet. Now is your chance to discover the right way, which is not as much about picking the perfect diet as it is about making a total commitment.

Why is changing your diet such a roller coaster ride of ups-and-downs and round-and-rounds? Because this isn't just a matter of changing the way you eat or exercise. It's a matter of transforming the way you think. The only way to succeed is to know beyond a shadow of a doubt that the discomfort you're suffering while you're working your weight loss program is far less than the discomfort you'll experience down the road, should you fail.

I've found that there are five levels of commitment.

The Five Levels of Commitment (More on this later):

1. A verbal declaration to yourself

2. A written declaration to yourself

3. A verbal declaration to another person

4. A written declaration to another person

5. A written declaration to another person with something to lose if you fail to perform.

Chapter 4

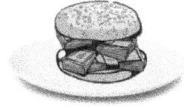

Raising the Stakes

You would think the stakes are already high enough to convince us to stay in shape. For those who are seriously overweight, the stakes can truly be life and death. If the existing stakes were absolute convincers, nobody would ever have trouble staying on a healthy diet. Maybe the stakes we're used to don't convince us because we know that everybody dies at some point, and the date of our death will always be an unknown. The kind of stakes that convince us to change our ways are those terrible certainties that we can create a way to avoid.

Let me introduce you to Rose and Kate, two typical dieters who tried to raise the stakes by finding a partner to diet with. Rose was a few pounds overweight and a couple of dress sizes too big for her body type. She had unhealthy eating habits and was unable to say no whenever sweet, rich goodies came her way. Exercise had become cumbersome. She resisted the idea of becoming the new fat person at the gym.

One day Rose's BFF, Kate, stopped by her house with news of the latest and greatest diet. She told Rose that if they took some new supplements, they could eat all their favorite foods and still lose weight. It sounded too good to be true. It was.

Luckily, Rose was smart enough to read the fine print on the bottle, which recommended she limit her calories. It also recommended being physically active. Okay. No problem. She no longer had to face this hurdle alone. Together, the girls joined a Curves fitness center. That was a super smart choice. The other members were mostly women at various levels of weight and fitness, so Rose and Kate did not feel ashamed of being overweight and enjoyed the support of other women. What's more, the facility had experts who provided much better information about what a healthy weight loss program really entailed.

Rose and Kate grew very excited about becoming hot looking and eye-catching again. The first week went great. After their workouts, the girls met at a health food store for lunch. Each was feeling better than she had in years. By the end of that week, some of the puffiness was already leaving their faces. The workouts felt good: not too fast, not too slow, but just right. They started to feel pretty again, not only on the outside, but also on the inside.

Back on Kate's home front, things were not so hunky dory. Kate's boyfriend, Chip, did not like all the veggies and broiled chicken thighs that began showing up on his dinner plate. There was no beer in the fridge. Kate was no longer excited about going out for pizza. Of course Chip wanted a hot girlfriend... Or did he? If Kate became super cute again, would she still want Chip for a boyfriend? He loved her, but he felt threatened. Chip started complaining. So Kate tried to please him.

Like a good little GF, Kate began shopping for two, not just in terms of quantity, but also variety: ground beef and beer for Chip, chicken and veggies for her; half-and-half for Chip's coffee, non-fat milk for hers. She grew resentful. When she reached the ice cream aisle, instead of buying Chip's favorite, she bought her own favorite flavor instead.

When she got home, the conflict escalated. "What kind of man eats cookie-dough ice cream?" Chip shouted at Kate.

"Where the hell is my rocky road with marshmallows in it?" Kate laughed under her breath, but the tension was building. They were not good at talking about their problems.

Chip stomped out to the bar for a beer with his bros. Kate broke down and ate the entire pint of Cookie Dough ice cream. Chip was not good at apologizing, so he just didn't come home that night. Kate felt so ashamed of the petty fight, and of cheating on her diet, that she actually craved more food to stop her emotional pain. At midnight, she began to worry that Chip wasn't coming home, so she popped some popcorn with melted butter. It did not make her feel better. By the next morning, she was angry that Chip never made it home. So when she poured her morning coffee, she added half-and-half, which looked much more soothing than the non-fat creamer.

By noon, it was time to go to Curves to work out with Rose. Kate went, but it was not as fun as it was the first week. She did not tell Rose about cheating on the diet, only that Chip was a jerk.

By the next night Chip came home. They got right down to making up. Chip even offered to take Kate out to a restaurant with plenty of healthy choices. This was great; except Kate was so relieved she was in a mood to celebrate, so she ordered the fish and chips. "At least it's fish," she justified her choice to herself.

Soon her weight loss plan turned into an ordeal. She was ashamed of cheating on her diet and ashamed of her inability to maintain an equitable relationship with her boyfriend. Instead of taking that as a cue to recommit to her program or work on asserting herself in her relationship, she ate her way deeper into her shame. She was not as pretty as she wanted, but at least the tension was gone in her relationship with chip. So was some of the passion. Her enthusiasm to be skinny again had vanished into the black hole of negativity that now clouded her whole diet. Oh well, at least she no longer had to deal with the effort it took to change her comfortable eating habits. Kate slipped right back into her comfort zone as if the diet had never happened.

Rose decided to try sticking to her diet without Kate. Kate felt ashamed that she had failed her friend, but the muffins at her favorite coffee place buried that shame, for a while. The two friends didn't see much of each other for a while because their paths had diverged. Rose was hanging at Curves and the health food store, while Kate was eating her shame at her comfortable old haunts.

The two met up again when Rose attended Chip's surprise birthday party. She felt obligated to "try" the cake since Kate had made it herself. To make up for indulging in cake, Rose stuck to the vegetable portion of the snack table, but she couldn't resist the ranch dip.

The next day, Rose felt disappointed with herself for breaking her diet. So she tried to make herself feel better by having a pastry with her usually healthy juice drink. That night, when she and her date went to a movie and he offered her popcorn, she figured she was already off-target for the day and asked for butter. They went out for a beer or two after the movie. Feeling like a failure, Rose gave up the diet, just a few weeks after Kate.

Rose and Kate are best of friends again. They sit on the sofa and talk. They eat what they want. They laugh about the time they tried that stupid diet and how it messed up their lives. Chip is happy again, kind of. At least, his fridge is stocked with beer and he knows noone will make a pass at Kate. Now *that's social security.*

Not exactly the happy ending you were hoping for is it?

Most of us overeaters try to eat our way out of fear and shame, only to end up eating our way into it. Eating gives us a momentary rush, like drugs or alcohol. The greatest thing, and the worst thing, about is that we can so easily justify it. After all, we have to eat to survive. Maybe we don't need the 5000-calorie all-you-can-eat buffet. But we cannot simply cut food out of our life, something we can do with drugs or alcohol. Once we open the door to food we need, it's easy to let a flood of food we don't need ride in with it.

Even though it helps alcoholics to use the buddy system of AA to get sober, sometimes the buddy system alone is not enough to get overeaters to cut back. We still have to eat, so when we hang out with friends who are easily tempted to go overboard, it's hard to know when or how to stop.

Yes, friends can help, but promises must be made in a way that breaking them is unthinkable.

Committing to Avoid the Unthinkable

The *Put Your Money Where Your Mouth Is* style of commitment uses the kind of leverage that will keep you on track. Shame or a sense of failure has sent you into a tailspin when you've cheated in the past. With my approach, you'll make an unbreakable commitment that will pull you out of the tailspin. Your promises to others—yes, it needs to be more than one—will create a force inside your mind that will not let you continue in your cycle of cheat-shame-cheat-shame-cheat.

Commitment-based dieting lets you cheat like a successful dieter. It lets you cheat like a pro.

Commitment-based dieting lets you cheat like a successful dieter. It lets you cheat like a pro. It gives you incentive, real incentive, not to cheat at all. When you do, because everybody does, you *will* find a way to course-correct. Maybe you'll hire a coach. Maybe you'll attend a support group for dieters. Maybe you'll decide that your commitment is just plain insufficient to accomplish your goals. Maybe you'll do what I did and get vitamin shots in your butt and some counseling for your head.

You might be thinking, "Dang Daniel, you make this system sound like a magic bullet." Not exactly. You still have to work at walking the precarious tight-rope of your diet, just as you did before, with a Level Five commitment you'll be working with a net. Nothing makes the world run as smoothly as commitment. Consider the house you live in. Is your rental agreement or your mortgage contract a magic bullet? Yes and No. On the surface, it's a standard agreement between you and another party. The scary magic is that this contract gives the other party the power to take away the roof over your head if you don't pay every month. The positive magic is that the potential consequence of failure forces you to keep your word. Maybe you've been late on a house payment during a really bad month, but it's the first bill you get back on track with immediately, because you don't want to lose your house.

That is the *magic bullet* of *Put Your Money Where Your Mouth Is*. When you cheat, you get caught up again pretty quick. If you want to make success at weight loss at least as likely as keeping your home, the most sure-fire way I've found is to create a contract with another human being that imposes high stakes for failure.

Sure, a handful of people can succeed at dieting without a high-stakes contract of some kind, but they are few and far between. They're probably not you, or you wouldn't be reading this.

One person I know found a way to create high stakes without a contract, but he didn't do so on purpose. It nearly killed him. My teacher Jeff looked death squarely in the face. He was a jock who let himself reach 90 pounds overweight. It didn't happen all at once, of course, but little by little. Being an athlete, he knew what was happening to his body. Being tough, he learned to live with it, little by little. His physical prowess got lost in his bad habits. Then he got the biggest wakeup call of all: BOOM, heart attack. It was a big one. It almost killed him.

It did not take him long to hire a professional coach, to do exactly what she said, to stay on course most of the time, and to get back on course whenever he strayed. Jeff shed the extra pounds the way he had gained them, little by little. He didn't just lose the weight. He gained his freedom. He gained a sense of accomplishment. He regained his self-confidence.

You and I don't have to have a heart attack kick us in the butt. We can create an unthinkable consequence for failure that won't kill us. Maybe it's not as motivating as staring death in the face. Wouldn't it be easier to create a commitment with consequences so dire you'll get on track before you end up with the unwanted motivation of a heart attack? This really is life and death; you just have to find another way to convince yourself.

With my commitment-based dieting strategy, you can manufacture your own consequences without having to go what Jeff went though. I've found that the fear of serious financial loss is as motivating for me as the fear of death was for Jeff. That is enough to stir up the same kind if determination in our primitive brain, the part of the brain that really calls the shots when we hit the fridge. Why wait until you end up like Jeff to set up some consequences that will get you moving? You can lose the weight starting now. All you need is an absolute commitment.

Food and Emotion

Food is emotional in one way or another for everybody. Emotions are like waves. If we don't get freaked out by them, they typically just pass. If we allow ourselves to feel our feelings, even when they hurt, then they too shall pass. If we resist our feelings because they're uncomfortable, we get stuck in an undertow and can't escape. Eating our way through our emotions is one way to resist them, and end up stuck in an undertow, turning over and over, drowning in the weight problem we've created because we couldn't face being sad, angry, lonely, inadequate, or bored.

On the surface, making a Level Five Commitment might seem to be all about weight, but it's also about returning harmony to your emotional life, so you can begin to find satisfaction in your total life. There is no emotion in the commitment itself. When you make a Level Five Commitment, you will send written pledges to several people, stating your measurable weight loss goal, the date by which you'll complete it, and the specific, major consequence you guarantee to pay if you fail. There shouldn't be any emotion in it, or you won't succeed. Yes, it will help you face your emotions and learn to live with them, because you have to. If you don't, if you start eating your way through your feelings, you're going to have to pay an unthinkable consequence, because you're not going to lose the weight.

Cheer up. With practice, you'll soon find the same thing that everyone who stops eating their feelings finds: you can survive your emotions.

Through this system you will be highly motivated to learn to swim or float through your negative feelings like a wave on the ocean. It might be powerful, but it is only passing. You'll break the habit of eating into your shame. You might even get far enough away from the shame to laugh at the pesky bugger.

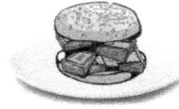

Chapter 5

All Diets Work If You Work Them

I'm a diet slut. I've lived with them all: Atkins, Zone, Fat Flush, Weight Watchers, Wheatgrass, fasting, and more. I would start out super excited. The foods and supplies were new. I had hope. Sometimes my friends were doing it too. Sometimes I'd already seen it work for them. Soon I began to lose weight. I was inspired!

Then life hit. An old friend from out of town showed up, or it was my brother's birthday, or I'd take my kids on vacation. I would put the program on hold. My commitment would grow weaker, while I would get fatter. Instead of taking the program off hold, I would just quit. I was tempted to blame the diet.

It's not the diets that are failing us.

A friend of mine did not get why I was talking about diets all the time. "Just eat healthy," she would say. She didn't understand my addiction issues because she'd never been around me when I was porky. She told me the popular adage, "Diets don't work." She was a *vegan*. I tried to tell her that vegan is a specific approach to eating, and is therefore a *diet*. It might be healthier than some of the diets I've tried, but it's still a diet.

It wasn't my diets that failed. It was me. It wasn't that the diet didn't work; it was that I didn't work the diet. The missing ingredient was not the right food or the right exercise, it was the right commitment. That's the only thing that will make a diet work.

An Addiction You Can't Quit

We all have to eat. Unfortunately, because our body needs sugar and fat for survival, we have a strong survival instinct to eat those two things. That craving probably worked wonders in motivating primitive humans to find and identify food sources, but today's ready-access to foods of all kinds has turned that natural craving against us.

Because we have to eat, sometimes staying on a healthy diet feels like living in a gray zone. It can be tricky to trust your instincts and the reptilian brain that runs them. When you make an unbreakable commitment to your goals for your body, you automatically enlist your higher-order brain, or neocortex, to help you. I have some news for your neocortex: it helps to stop looking at this as a battle between dieting and cheating, and instead look at each meal in terms of *away* versus *toward*. For instance fried chicken moves you *away* from your goals, while a plateful of vegetables moves you *toward* your goals.

If you're a food addict, you cannot just quit, unlike a smoker, alcoholic, or drug addict. You have to eat. This isn't about quitting, but about making a thousand little yes/no choices every day. How do you know when to say "yes" and when to say "no?" You really do need a diet plan. One way to make your diet fail is to look at it as the "law". Instead, look at your diet as a guideline. The only "law" is your commitment to pay if you don't let the guidelines *take you to your goal.*

Written dietary guidelines are what will take you from the dieting gray zone into black-and-white. Your guidelines tell you which eating decisions are taking your toward your goal and which are taking you away from it.

Chapter 6

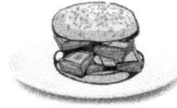

The Five Levels of Commitment

We have all had different experiences with commitment. To many people, it reflects something negative, a surrender of some aspect of ourselves or what we want. To others, the word is a positive gateway to the challenges that create opportunities for positive exchanges with others and positive changes for ourselves. A commitment can be as simple as the agreement to exchange cash for food. A commitment can be as complex as a company's promise to create a new product. The most successful people in the world are adept at making and keeping commitments.

Commitments make the world go 'round. They foster the relationships big and small that keep individuals, families, communities, and countries working together for the greater good. They keep society from falling into chaos. The commitments that people tend to keep are either those that don't take much effort, or those in which the stakes are too high to fail. Everyone knows that losing weight takes effort, so a commitment to lose weight is going to be hard to keep unless you raise the stakes. You need to understand the power of this tool. A commitment is not a diet. It is the lever you must pull to give yourself the surefire guarantee that you will follow through, maintain, and succeed at your diet. Commitments are made with a vision in mind. You want a certain outcome. So you declare what you want to accomplish, and you promise to do so. That's a commitment.

Not all commitments are created equal.
If you want to keep a commitment, you have
to learn how to guarantee it in a way that
leaves no room to back out.

The Five Levels of Commitment

For the purposes of a program like this one, we can break down the concept of commitment into five levels. Each level has its benefits, but each succeeding level offers a more powerful commitment than the one preceding it. The levels are:

1. **Verbal commitment to yourself.**

2. **Written commitment to yourself.**

3. **Verbal commitment to another person.**

4. **Written commitment to another person.**

5. **Written commitment to another person, with something to lose if you fail.**

Level 1: Verbal commitment to yourself

A Level One Commitment is a verbal commitment to yourself. You think hundreds of thousands of thoughts every day. The problem is, if you think about losing weight over and over again, that may feel like a commitment, but there is no accountability. Thoughts disappear without a trace, and nobody is the wiser. If you voice your promise aloud to yourself, maybe even in the mirror, that's a little more convincing. You might say, "I'm going to the gym today." The problem is, if you don't keep your word to yourself, there are no consequences. You can forget these words as easily as a passing breeze. Maybe you're about to grab your gym bag when you remember an email you have to send or the phone rings. Maybe a work problem needs solving or your friends invite you over. It's easy to decide, "Work comes first," or "Maintaining my friendships are important... I'll put off going to the gym until tomorrow." That thought makes just as much sense as the thought you had before.

Most people who go on diets never go beyond a Level One Commitment. It's that level of commitment that makes us feel out of control at times. It was the Level One Commitment that allowed me to become an expert in almond croissants. Used to be if I saw an almond croissant, a little voice in my head would say, "You're not eating almond croissants today." However, if the coffee line in front of the almond croissants took too long to move, another voice in my head would chime in with a completely different thought, "You should try that almond croissant. After all, you are an almond croissant connoisseur. I'll bet it's really good!" That voice sounds so pleasant, so agreeable, so understanding of my needs. So I order my coffee with the almond croissant. The saddest part is that it's usually not as good as I thought it was going to be. Five minutes later, my appetite is just as unsatisfied as it was when I was standing in line. If I eat another one, it's not going to be as good as the first. It never is. What was the point of all that?

If you want to make a commitment with some power, you have to be accountable to somebody besides the little voices in your head. Many Eastern religions focus on getting people to stop reacting to those thoughts. We have about 750,000 of them per day. They're never going to shut up. So how do you stop reacting? Meditation helps. As a Kundalini yoga instructor, I teach the use of mantra to quiet down that little voice in my head.

Nothing can make that head drivel stop forever. So if you want to arm yourself against its seductive sales pitches involving almond croissants, or whatever your weakness is, then I suggest increasing your level of commitment.

Level 2: Written Commitment to Yourself

At this level you have a thought and you take the time to write it down. Some examples of a Level Two Commitment might be: a promise made to yourself in a journal, a set of goals you've written on a sheet of notepaper, or an appointment you've entered into your personal calendar. It might even be a single line of affirmation on a scrap that you carry in your wallet.

The fact that you've written this thought down so that you can refer back to it at a later time gives you a higher degree of accountability. The problem is that you are the only person you're accountable to. Nobody else will know whether you succeed or fail because you haven't told them.

Self-accountability can still help in achieving small, interim goals on the way to your larger goals. It's not as if you can report to another person on everything you plan to do all day long. I've found that it helps to keep a calendar with a list of what I want to get done for that day. When I get all those items done, I get the satisfaction of marking a big black X through that day on the calendar. This is also a way of rooting myself on to success. If my goal is to lose a pound a week, and today I had a goal to hit the gym, then crossing that goal off my list is a way of telling myself, "Way to go, Daniel! You're on your way." It helps.

There are no real consequences for failure. So, once again, it's just too easy to simply say, "Oh well, I'll just move today's to-do item to tomorrow." For a person with food addiction issues, this is a major obstacle.

Level 3: Verbal commitment to another person

A Level Three Commitment requires you to make a verbal promise to one or more friends. If you make that promise to one person, you're in a partnership. If you make it to more than one person, *you're in a network*. In either case, you've gotten your community involved. We humans do better in a team than on our own, just as dolphins who hunt in pods and wolves who hunt in packs. It's often easier to accomplish hard tasks when we work with others.

A verbal commitment to another person is stronger than a written commitment to yourself, especially if you're not the kind of person who does whatever you say you're going to do. When you tell other people about your goals, you're more accountable for achieving them. Now your pride is on the line, if nothing else. You've added the element of bolstering your reputation by being a person of your word, or facing shame or embarrassment if you don't keep your word. If you tell the kinds of friends who are good at keeping you honest by telling you the hard truth, it sure helps. They become, in effect, your accountability team. The problem is that most people empathize with the difficulties of dieting. They're not going to blame you if you fail.

The most obvious weakness of a verbal commitment is the lack of clear consequences. Nobody's going to blame you if you don't lose the weight.

Usually, Level Three Commitments are pretty casual. When most people make a Level Three Commitment it happens by chance. Jill and Steph are chatting about a cool new diet that helped some movie star take off twenty pounds.

Your friend says something offhand like, "I could stand to lose twenty pounds."

Then you say, "I'm going to do it. I'm going to commit to lose twenty pounds in the next two months!"

Even better, maybe your friend chimes in, "I'll do it with you!"

"This will be fun!" you say.

It is… for at least the first week. Then something happens: a party, a bad day at work, or a spouse bringing home leftover cookies from the break-room. It's hard not to cheat. After you cheat the first time, it gets easier to cheat again. What's worse, your friend, the one you were counting on to keep you in line, thinks it's hard too. If you give up, you know she'll forgive you, and maybe even be relieved. Even if she never joined you in the diet in the first place, you know she'll understand. After all, she's your friend!

Making a Level Three Commitment, a verbal commitment to another person, can be a strong choice for some things: like planning a party, a date, or dinner with a friend. It's a weak choice for the big-ticket items: like buying a house, closing a business deal, or losing weight.

When it comes to dieting, social expectations are not high to begin with. If you're telling someone about yourself and what you've been up to, and you say, "I swear to you that I'm going to lose 10 pounds in two months." The other person probably doesn't see that statement as a commitment. To them it's just a casual conversation. It's possible they think you're just dreaming.

I have a friend who often tells me she's going to Italy someday. I believe her, because she's the type who follows through on what she speaks. When will she go? Who knows! Meanwhile, I have other friends who say the same sort of thing, and I think, "Yeah? I'll believe it when I see the ticket." I know they're just engaging in wishful thinking. They're not really planning. They're not determined. In either case, if they didn't make the trip, I wouldn't blame them. They don't owe me, or anyone, an explanation.

The Level Three Commitment is even weaker when it comes to weight loss, because if we tell people we're going to lose weight and we fail, that can cause the shame that leads us back to overeating. If we get embarrassed enough, we might spend a few nights raiding the ice cream in the fridge, and end up even heavier than we were before we started. A Level Three Commitment is just not strong enough to keep you steady when your emotions are swirling and your survival instincts are shouting for more food.

I still believe Level Three Commitments have an important place in your diet plan, but only as one piece of the puzzle. It's like a wedding vow. When people get married, they exchange vows in front of witnesses. In this ceremonial sense, that is a very powerful Level Three Commitment. Most couples don't stop there. They also get a marriage license, which adds a written component to back up the verbal.

The verbal component is important because it's a public declaration. If you break the commitment, people will know. The written component helps seal the deal, making your verbal promises undeniable before the law. You are now bound to stick to what you said. At the time, you might not be thinking about the consequences for failing to keep your promises. They're there. I promise you; they're there.

I don't suggest stopping at a Level Three Commitment. You might as well be planning to fail.

Level 4: Written commitment to another person

This is a written commitment between you and another person. This is more effective than a verbal commitment. A Level Four commitment is when you not only write it down, but you send it out to another person. In the old days, this was a letter or a postcard. Now, any email or text will do. For example, "I'm super excited because I have decided to lose 20 pounds in the next ninety days." As you can see, this is powerful because there is a written record of your declaration.

With social media, Level Four commitments become even stronger. You could post on Facebook that you will lose 20 pounds in 90 days. You would get back a good deal of support, advice, and most importantly accountability. Same goes for Twitter and even Snap Chat.

Words spoken disappear almost as quickly as thoughts. Words can be forgotten, misinterpreted, not remembered correctly, or just plain *denied*. "I never said *that! What I said was...*" As the old Texas saying goes, "If it ain't written, it ain't true."

Nobody likes *looking bad* in front of other people so now the pressure is on. You went public. You came out of the closet. You made a public declaration. You are beginning to get reptilian brain on your side because looking bad in front of the tribe could mean being ostracized, kicked out: probable death. The reptilian brain will go to great measures to avoid these calamities. When you make a public declaration, reptilian brain listens. Not bad!

Level 5: Written commitment to another person, with something to lose if you fail

This is a written commitment between you and another person, in which you promise to do something specific, for which there is a penalty for failure to perform. It's the kind of commitment that builds skyscrapers and great ships at sea. It's the kind of commitment that builds companies like Google and Apple. A Level Five commitment turns your word into your bond. You cannot afford to break your word because there could be dire consequences for breaking what is, technically, a contract.

It's usually easiest to make the price too high if it's a financial one, but you can also give up something else, so long as it has the power to make failure not an option. Promise them your boat, your favorite painting, your wine collection, whatever. Just make sure it's something you can't bear the thought of losing. That doesn't mean you should put your life savings in jeopardy, but there's plenty of potential pain available under that mark.

The promise needs to engage your reptilian brain with fear that it might have a harder time surviving with the penalty than living without the sugary, fatty foods it wants all the time.

Bankers and landlords already know the power of a Level Five Commitment. They know that if you fail to pay the mortgage or the rent on time, they can foreclose on your house or evict you. Bankers and landlords always operate in Level Five Commitments: always in writing, and always with a penalty.

When I rented the space for my Mexican Taqueria, the commercial landlords wanted to be able to evict me not only from my restaurant if I did not pay the rent buy from my home as well. This was great leverage for them, because they knew that protecting one's home is a top priority for most people. This is why banks and landlords always get paid first. They know we're motivated not to lose our houses. If you want to make big things happen in your life, a Level Five Commitment is the way to go.

Dr. Donald Hensrud, editor of the *Mayo Clinic Diet*, conducted a study that included 100 employees of the clinic. The participants either received a $20 reward if they reached their monthly weight loss goals, or were penalized $20 if they failed. Another group received no financial incentive at all. Of the participants who were given a cash incentive, 62% lost weight. Meanwhile only 26% of those who received no cash incentive succeeded at losing weight. "This could be one piece of the puzzle to help people achieve their healthy weight goals," said Dr. Hensrud.

I think it's significant to note that the subjects did not have that much money to gain or lose in Dr. Hensrud's experiment. It doesn't take much for most people to respond positively to the external pressure of the wager, although for a stubborn guy like me it takes a mountain. "Financial incentives and disincentives can help people lose weight, and keep it off for one year," said Dr. Steven Driver, resident physician in internal medicine at the Mayo Clinic in Rochester, Minnesota. "It's not about getting rich, it's about being held accountable."

The Mayo Clinic study demonstrates the power of a Level Five commitment: a commitment in writing, to another person or institution, in which you have something to gain or lose should you fail.

Losing weight is one of the most difficult things you'll ever do, and it ultimately is a life or death proposition. Yet there's a lot of emotional baggage and bodily instinct wrapped up in keeping you overweight. It takes the highest level of commitment to make that kind of change. Level Five: between you and another person, in writing, with a promise to pay big for failure.

A Level Five Commitment closes the back door, so you can't simply escape when the going gets tough. A Level Five Commitment gets you out of your head. The question of "if" is gone. You no longer wonder "if" you're going to lose weight. One way or another, you are going to lose it.

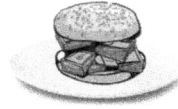

Chapter 7

Choosing Your Diet

The word *diet* is going out of style. People are disillusioned and hurt by the results from complicated and sometimes high-tech ways of solving an age old problem. "Diet" originally meant what we eat. What you put in your mouth is your diet. What you put in your mouth should be healthy. There will always be debate over what that means.

Here's what I've discovered about diets in the sense of programs to lose weight: All diets work, even the ridiculous or unhealthy ones. I'm not saying they'll all make you healthy and fit. If you change the way you eat, and you stick with it, it will change your body. It's simple math. If you consume fewer calories than you expend, you will lose weight. Don't let yourself fall in the trap of blaming the diet. In fact, your commitment shouldn't let you.

Plenty of smart people have created a variety of healthy programs to make it as easy as possible to lose weight. You still have to do the work. If you're following the program and it's not working, then the answer isn't to blame the diet, but to eat a little less or exercise a little more. If that doesn't help, keep adjusting. If that still doesn't help, maybe you've chosen an unwise diet, but that still doesn't let you off the hook. It's up to you to switch to a diet that does work. You're responsible for your diet. Your diet is not responsible for you.

There's no way around the fact that success is more about the commitment to the diet than it is about the diet itself. This isn't about the diet, it's about you. When I say "all diets work," I'm saying that they work if you're committed.

So how do you choose a diet? If a friend at work recommends a diet and says that it worked great for her, should you try it? If you have some confidence in it, ask your doctor what he or she thinks. If there's no medical reason that it could be bad for you, go for it!

If you spend a week on your new diet and realize you can't face this style of eating for the rest of your life, you might want to try another healthy option. If you spend several weeks on it and your weight doesn't budge, then definitely try something else. Either way, you will find a way to hit your weight goal, because you've made a commitment to do so and you're going to have to pay until it hurts if you don't.

That's why you must make a specific commitment, in writing, to more than one person, with a promise of dire consequences for failure. Otherwise, you're putting the diet in the driver's seat, when it's your commitment itself that must be in charge.

I'm not going to pick your diet. Have you chosen a healthy diet? That I cannot say. Have you accidentally chosen a diet that burns muscle instead of fat? That I cannot say. Will you put the weight right back on after you get it off? Not if you make a new commitment immediately upon getting it off. That I cannot say. Will your diet work for you? If you are committed enough, you will find a diet that works for you. Finding the diet that you like best is up to you. I'm just saying that it's the commitment that will make the diet work, no matter which diet you choose.

Consulting a doctor before starting any kind of diet program is important. In terms of succeeding at your diet, it's critical that you pick an approach you believe in. Whatever goes into your selection process, if you have confidence that you'll lose weight on the program you chose, then half the battle is already won. The other side of that coin is true as well: if you think a particular weight loss program is a bunch of rubbish, then it probably won't work for you.

The diet just gives you the tools. Those tools might include a certain caloric intake, certain kinds of food, certain drinks, certain supplements, and an exercise routine. You must wield those tools with total commitment or it won't work. The urge to cheat is human, primitive, and strong. So your commitment can't just be an idea or concept. It must be a contract.

One important thing to remember is that if your diet gives you tools and if you have a commitment to make those tools work, then you had better find out how to use them properly. In other words: follow your diet's instructions. You can't just follow one part of the plan and not another, or keep changing the rules to suit your mood.

Is there a perfect diet out there for you? Yes and no. The perfect diet will be the one that you feel most confident in. The perfect diet will keep you from losing the money you've pledged. Don't beat yourself up for where you are. That might be how you got there. Be easy on yourself. This time, when you make a decision to lose weight, stop trying to rely on willpower alone, and allow yourself to lean on something else. Cut yourself a break and make a commitment… or three.

What will you lean on? *An unbreakable commitment.* Almost any diet you pick will work, so long as the consequence for failure is a price you cannot easily afford. If your diet truly isn't working, you'll know pretty quickly. The reality of facing severe consequences will tell you whether you're just making excuses or really need a different diet. Don't be afraid to change boats mid-stream if absolutely necessary.

Since this is more about the commitment than the weight loss program itself, don't agonize over the program you choose: Weight Watchers, Overeaters Anonymous Blood Type diet, South Beach diet, low-fat, low-carb, no sugar, residential treatment, the gym, whatever. Just pick an approach and get a move on!

Why Diets Work

Ideally what a weight loss program is supposed to do is cause your body to burn off its fatty storage. Beyond that, there's a quagmire of theories about which kind of fat you should burn, how the liver is involved, whether a particular program burns fat or muscle or just dumps excess water. The medical community is working night and day to end this obesity problem and create functioning diets.

Since our bodies store fat as a reserve for hungrier times, we have to trick our bodies into believing that these are the hungry times. Our bodies need to burn more fat then they store. If we do this improperly, it feels like starvation, as if we're stranded on a desert island. If we go at this too aggressively, we can make ourselves weak, spacey, tired, empty, and forlorn. Who in their right mind wants to feel that bad?

Finding the right approach for you comes down to basic body chemistry. You must find the right combination of eating and exercise habits that get your body's chemical wonderland to send signals to the fat storage cells that it's okay to stop holding on to that fat for dear life.

You might be thinking, "Wow, Daniel, you seem to have more faith in modern weight loss plans than most of my fat friends. If they work so well, then why is obesity the biggest health issue in America today?" *Commitment.* No matter how good the program you pick, it's going to require you to change your lifestyle. Losing weight is uncomfortable, both physically and emotionally. Changing your eating habits may be one of the most difficult things you'll ever do. That takes discipline.

Accountability

If you've made a Level Five Commitment—to more than one person, in writing, detailing specific goals, and a painful penalty for failure—then you have a much better chance of picking a diet that will truly bring you success. In my opinion, the best weight loss programs ask you to write down all you consume, the hours you work out, and the important physical changes involved—usually weight loss, but maybe inches, body fat, blood sugars, or other measurements. This alone will go a long way to keep you on track.

Keeping your commitment is about accountability. If you get on the scale every day, write down the results, and create a weekly graph, you'll be much more motivated not to cheat. You'll have a much more constant eye on how far you're moving toward or away from your goal.

Nobody said this would be easy. Change is hard. You probably won't like it at first. When you get on a roll and your diet starts working for you, you'll find a balance between weight loss and discomfort. Then you will feel empowered. After a while it will become easier, like everything else you ever became good at. If you run six flights of stairs every day to get to your office, at first you might be out of breath, but after a week, you'll notice that it's a little easier. And after a few weeks, you might even realize that it's barely any more effort than crossing a street. After a month or two, you might even be eager for a harder challenge.

This is a step-by-step process. Break your goal into little chunks. If your ultimate goal is to lose fifty pounds, and you dwell on that number every day, you're going to make yourself nuts the first time you hit the scale and only see one pound gone. That kind of frustration can drive people to cheat. Consider thinking in terms of a pound or two a week, or five to ten pounds a month. Don't plan to lose everything all at once.

Don't plan to lose weight too fast either. Take your time. It probably took you years to get out of shape, so it might take you at least a few months to get back into shape. It probably took you years to get entrenched in your bad habits, so give yourself time to develop new habits that you can sustain in the coming years.

After you make a public declaration and back it up by sending written commitments to people who you know will hold your feet to the fire, you will have an instant support group. You are accountable to these people in more ways than one. You have promised that if you fail you' will give them something important to you. You might have promised to give them money, or to do something embarrassing. Maybe you're a devoted member of a political party and you promised to donate $3000 to the opposing party if you failed to reach your goal-weight. Maybe you made that promise to four people, for a total of $1200! Now that would get you motivated!

Although it's definitely important to pick a definite diet and fitness plan, complete with guidelines, you should not start your diet until after you make your Level Five Commitments. Here's the basic order I recommend doing things in, 1) set a realistic goal, 2) set a timetable that includes a couple of weeks at the front to pick a diet, and perhaps a couple of weeks at the end to give yourself some padding, 3) send out your pledges.

I don't recommend starting your diet until *after* you send your written pledges, complete with consequences, to at least three people. Four is better. If you know yourself to have trouble with accountability, five is even better. The reason to send the pledges first is so that you don't start the diet until after your commitment is in place. The commitment is what will set your diet in motion and keep it going.

When dieting, put the horse before the cart.
The commitment is the horse, the diet is the cart.

Chapter 8

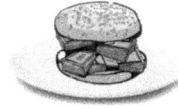

Commitment, The Missing Link

When I first made the commitment to lose weight, I didn't put enough money where my mouth was to keep it off. The incentive I created wasn't big enough for me to fear the pain of losing money more than I feared the pain of missing out on caramel ice cream and sugary peanut butter. So I had to up the ante. I sent out three new pledges to friends with astronomical price tags for failure. As soon as I sent those, I knew I needed a plan that I was not going to wriggle out of so easily. I made an appointment with an intensive weight loss clinic that specialized in offering a food-cleanse diet and supplements.

The new program made a lot more sense to me than what I had been doing before. The healthy and beautiful women who helped me at the clinic verified that I had been eating too much sugar, a common problem for alcoholics. Of course, if I'd really thought about it before, it would have been obvious to me. What helped me stop living in denial were the dollar signs in my new pledges: I couldn't afford not to see the truth.

If I had just gone to the clinic without laying some serious money on the line beforehand, I might easily have let the expert advice slip in one ear and out the other. I might have slacked off on following the diet to cleanse my system, or forgotten to take the supplements.

Sending the commitments out first is what made me get real about it when I walked into that clinic. Suddenly I felt hope and clarity where before I'd known only shame and bewilderment.

Don't think that just because you've checked into an expensive spa or residency program, you can therefore afford to forego sending out your unbreakable pledges to your accountability partners. Residency programs can help you set and achieve short term goals. They can work with you on reprogramming the way you eat and creating new habits. They can offer counseling and support groups to help you deal with the emotional roots of your overeating. Those are all great things. They will not substitute for having something major to lose if you should fail.

You see, although you might make a financial investment to a residency program, they're keeping that money whether you succeed or fail. With your accountability partners, you only have to pay if you fail—and the amount will be punishing, because you'll promise to make it punishing. That is an incentive so scary it makes your commitment unbreakable.

Don't be afraid of making the commitment outrageously expensive. The higher the cost of failure, the less likely you are to get stuck in a cheating cycle. Better to risk your money on your health than to risk dying fat and young.

Your high-priced commitment tells your reptilian brain that you're going to succeed. Your pledges shout to your friends that you are $300 or $3000 or $3 million (Donald Trump) sure that you will succeed. *Your pledge has to hurt so much that you truly believe you have no option to fail.* You can't let fear of failure convince you to make a small pledge, or this is never going to work. These pledges can't be empty gestures. They have to be real promises with real financial or sentimental weight.

You don't need to pay for some fancy health resort to weight. If you don't have a lot of money to burn, that makes this commitment even easier. You don't have to promise a lot to make the consequences too big for you to fail. In the long run, the guy who can only afford to promise three $100 pledges and buy a cheap book on healthy eating and a pair of workout shoes has an advantage over the guy who can afford time and money for a health resort but doesn't leverage his commitment with something tangible to lose.

The low-budget guy with pledges will lose weight within the parameters of his world, because he has given himself no choice. He'll have an incentive for creating strategies on how to get through birthday parties or Friday donuts at work. He'll have the greater motivation for toughing out the lonely late-night hours when it's just him and his beloved fridge. Maybe he'll find a cheap 12-step group like Overeaters Anonymous, or he'll start hanging out with skinny friends. Meanwhile, the guy at the health resort has already spent his money before he even lost the weight. He has nothing else to lose. When the going gets tough, what's his incentive to keep going?

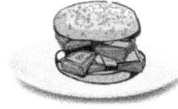

Chapter 9

Making Your Level Five Commitment

If you really want to succeed at this, then you'll need to send your Level Five Commitments, or pledges, to at least three people. The moment they receive those pledges, those three people will become your accountability team. It's still possible one person might flake out and decide to let you off the hook at the last minute, but never all three.

Whatever you choose to give up, just remember Daniel's Golden Rule: "If you're not feeling motivated, than you have not committed enough gold."

Making your Level Five Pledges shouldn't be complicated. In fact, it will work best if you keep it simple. You enroll the other parties in your Level Five Commitment simply by writing them an email stating your goal weight and your goal date. In the document, you promise that if you don't reach that weight by that date, you will give that person X number of dollars. Make sure the chunk of money you specify is a whopper. If you want you can also agree to give up your boat, your prized stamp collection, your baseball signed by Babe Ruth, that you'll do something embarrassing like streaking or any creative combination of these things (whatever motivates you to truly believe failure is not an option). Tell them that the verification will be a text or email of a photo of your feet on a scale with the goal weight clearly visible.

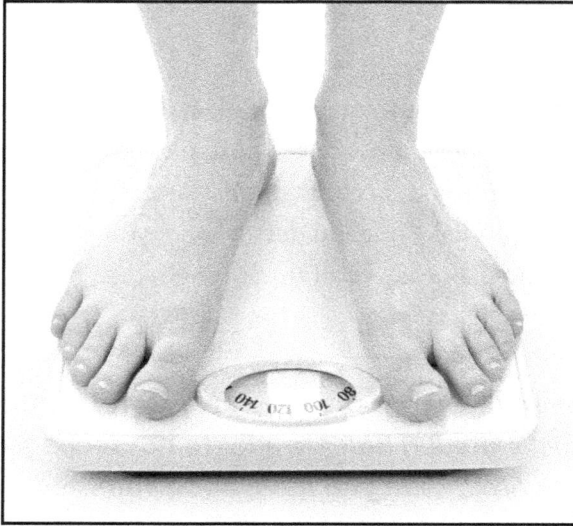

Why go through this alone any longer? *Type up those pledges and email them.* Your pledges don't need to be more than a couple of lines. For example: "Dear Jackie, I promise to reach my goal weight of 172 pounds (or less) by June 1, 2015. If I don't reach that weight by that date, I will pay you $1000 the next day and run through downtown Phoenix underwear. I will text/email you a photo of my feet on the scale when I succeed. Thanks for your support in this endeavor."

That's all you need. Your new life starts the moment you hit the SEND key.

Your Pledges Create Momentum and Support

You may notice an interesting feeling after you hit SEND on those three emails, or drop those three envelopes in the mailbox: That feeling is certainty. You realize now that you have no choice but to succeed. You have sent out a ticking time bomb that will explode if you fail, taking with it an unbearable sum of your life savings (or whatever else you decided you couldn't bear to lose).

By sending out your Level Five pledges, you turn inertia into momentum, thereby turning fear into action. In the past, you felt uncertain about whether you could stick to your diet or whether the diet would work for you. At some point, uncertainty led you to hesitate, balk, and give up. You ended up stuck in the mud, unable to move.

When you send out your pledges, you feel the inertia giving way to the current of a new tide. That current carries you. You're so full of clear, confident certainty that new ideas begin to reveal themselves to you, and supportive people begin to show up for you. Your confidence attracts what you need to succeed. Your pledges create a momentum that carries you in the direction of beauty. This momentum will sweep you off your feet. Let it. It's an exhilarating ride.

"…the moment one definitely commits oneself, then Providence moves too."
– William Hutchison Murray

Pledges have another fantastic effect, aside from making you accountable to other people. They also turn other people into your support group. You think your friends want to take your money in this little wager? No, that would not be a "win" for them. Instead, it would put them in the awkward position of gaining at your expense. Now that they know how much it means to you to succeed, and what you're willing to put on the line, they're going to back you up. There's nothing like the power of friendship, harnessed tightly to a dream. What I'm saying is: you're no longer alone in this struggle.

Maybe you're thinking, "I don't get it, Daniel. The last time I checked, dieting was a solo game. I'm responsible for my own body and mind, right? I'm the one eating the veggies instead of the bacon, right?" Yes and no. Indeed you're the only one who will suffer the physical consequences of gaining or losing weight, not your doctors, not your insurance company, not your friends, nor the government. Nobody can force you to put anything in your mouth, except you.

If you Google "diet betting" online, you'll discover there are now plenty of places to bet on yourself in the cyber community. I don't recommend that method. The problem is that those bets are secret. Sure, it gives you a financial incentive. It doesn't create a tribe of supporters. It doesn't require anyone who cares about you to know that you're on a diet. You can go online with a fake username and bet against somebody in Madagascar or Brazil, and if you fail you lose a couple hundred bucks. Big deal.

The cyber-betting world is missing out on leveraging one important feature of your reptilian brain. The reptilian brain fears the loss of status that can come from failing to complete a task in front of a community of witnesses. Yes, the reptilian brain also hates to lose money, but not as much as it hates to look bad.

That's why it's more powerful to make these agreements with people you personally know.

By creating other consequences and involving your *friends* in those consequences, you can create an aspect of dieting that is no longer just about your health. If you can do that effectively, you're no longer in this alone. With your pledges you change the stakes of the diet game. You increase the stakes for yourself, and invite other teammates to share the stakes with you. It might seem as if you're playing against each other, but actually you're on the same side.

This is a win-win situation. If you succeed, you'll be healthier and happier, and they'll be happy for you. If you fail, they won't go down with you, but will instead receive compensation for playing. For them it's a win-win. And if you do this right, it's a win-win for all of you. If you make the price of failure high enough, neither you nor they will let you fail. None of you wants that.

These pledges create a new harmony between you and your accountability partners. You've laid all the cards on the table. Each party knows what they have to do to assist the other. It's a win-win situation. Now you have three more people working with you to achieve the same goal. They are rooting for you. If you need them to talk you through a rough spot, police your refrigerator, or go with you to the gym, one of those three people is more likely to help.

The more people you enlist to support you, the easier, and more fun, it will be to work toward your goal. You're going to get there no matter what—but there's no reason to be miserable along the way, when you can always enlist your friends to join your support team and cheer you on.

Put Your Money Where Your Mouth Is

Your Commitment Creates Self-Confidence

You know that feeling of excitement when you know something great is about to happen? Something you want, something you've been dreaming about, something you have been yearning for. The day you realize that it's all up to you and you have the key in your hand is the day you begin to taste the triumph that is inevitably coming your way. Maybe what you're looking forward to is you dream house, a luxury car, or your wedding day. Or maybe it's the day you step on the scale and the number returns to what it was when you were 25. Whatever it is, when you have the power to make big things happen, and you finally take the step that you are certain will set you on your way to attain it, you feel the call to action.

When you have been thinking about, talking about, and wondering about a decision for days, months, or years, there's a very real change in energy that takes place when you finally make the decision. Your body is simultaneously supercharged with energy and relaxed with certainty. "Ahhhhh…" Because once you do that one thing that you know is going to make it all work, you realize that although attainment may take more work than you've ever done before, you've also made it easier than ever before to do that work—without needing to worry about whether it's all going to work out. That's the great thing about a Level Five Commitment: it has taken all the guess-work out of this. You're on the road to what you want and there's no turning back.

As you send out your three written pledges to friends, promising to lose weight or pay big, you don't even need to worry that this is the first time you've made a Level Five Commitment. It's not. You are an experienced Level Five Committer.

It's how you got your education, your car, your home, your marriage, your business, your phone, or any other major life change or purchase you've committed to. If you've ever taken a vacation to a dream destination, you even purchased that privilege with a Level Five Commitment. Those plane tickets were nonrefundable, weren't they?

I'm always excited and nervous right after I purchase an airplane ticket, because I know for sure that I'm going somewhere. That's how it feels to make your Level Five Commitment to lose weight.

Think about the last time you signed a document to make a big commitment. Did you pause for just a moment to let the import of what you were doing sink in? Did you feel butterflies in your belly? Were you excited and scared at the same time? Those final questions run through your head. What if it doesn't work out? What if something changes and I can't live up to these terms? What if I change my mind? After you sign, even though the excitement remains, all the nervous what-ifs suddenly vanish, and you relax into the knowledge that you are strapped in and heading on the ride to your dream.

Chapter 10

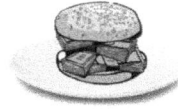

Loss is Stronger Than Gain

W hy does a Level Five Commitment guarantee you'll lose weight, when Levels One through Four do not? Why aren't all the benefits of living a healthy, long, slender life enough to motivate us to create it?

It's human nature to be more motivated by the possibility of losing something you have, than by the possibility of gaining something you never had in the first place.

The rewards of losing weight at some foggy future point can seem too nebulous to us in the moment. We can barely imagine the pleasures of slenderness in the face of a low blood sugar craving for pie and ice cream. However, the fear of losing money and pride can terrify us into doing whatever it takes right now. We hate to lose what we have more than we are willing to strive for what we can hardly conceive.

Humans will always fight much harder to protect what they have then to risk losing for future gain. That's true, even when what they have to gain is of greater value. In other words, people hate to lose more than they love to win.

This syndrome is known as *loss aversion*. It was first demonstrated by Amos Tversky and Daniel Kahneman. Loss aversion is a central premise in the *Put Your Money Where Your Mouth Is* commitment-based diet concept. Some studies suggest that fear of loss is twice as powerful, psychologically, as the desire for gain.

Another study documented in *Good Housekeeping* magazine found that "Dieters who stood to lose money if they didn't succeed in shedding weight were about five times as likely to reach their goals as those with no financial stake in the outcome."

So, with the *Put Your Money Where Your Mouth Is* plan, we look for ways to leverage our fears. The fear of losing face is a huge motivator. A Level Five Commitment takes advantage of that. If you fail, people will know. Then, to add insult to injury, you add the fear of losing your money or possessions. These potential losses are highly motivating because your reptilian brain hates to lose. That part of your nervous system will work very hard not to lose. The primitive in you may not want to step out of his comfort zone to win a healthy body, but he will step out of his comfort zone to protect his precious clutch of eggs from being taken away.

The best thing about a Level Five Commitment is that there's no way out.

If you can find a way out of your commitment, then it wasn't a Level Five Commitment, and you need to reset. With a Level Five Commitment, you have to give yourself so much to lose that you will do anything—within the law of course—to prevent that.

Chapter 11

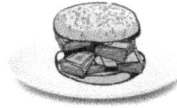

Commitment Overcomes Obstacles

Making an unbreakable commitment doesn't mean you will eliminate obstacles. Instead, the commitment is what gives you the strength to overcome the obstacle. The commitment doesn't make battling obstacles easy, only necessary. Necessity is the mother of invention. If you know that you don't have the option to quit in the face of adversity because the consequences are too great, then you're not going to quit. The commitment forces you to find the limits of your own strength. You'll discover they're greater than you imagined.

When you decide to make a real lasting change in your life, like losing weight, resistance is normal. Change is not easy. You and your body aren't going to like it at first.

A strong commitment helps us move through moments of resistance.

The beauty of a strong commitment is the power it has to move us through resistance. "An object at rest tends to stay at rest, while an object in motion tends to stay in motion" (–Sir Isaac Newton.) Sometimes we're stuck at rest, or our momentum is taking the scale in the wrong direction. We realize we have to get off our butts and move, or change our eating habits so we can move the scale the other way. Our commitment is our own self-appointed parent who stands over us and says, "You better, or else…here's the punishment I have in store for you!" "Oh, right," you remember, "I'm going to lose my shirt if I don't take off this weight. I'd better change something I'm doing, fast!"

"Neither snow, nor rain, nor heat, nor gloom of night stays these couriers from swift completion of their appointed rounds." (–James Farley on the wall of the NYC post office.)

An unbreakable commitment is capable of assuring you get the task done no matter what obstacles you face along the way.

Success Has Its Privileges

Thanks to a Level Five Commitment, I have lost my spare tire and am now working on my six-pack. Once the Level Five Commitment strapped me in without the option to fail, I had fun with it. I've found that the Level Five Commitment is such a powerful tool, that sometimes I find it too much a hassle to get anything done until I've made that supercharged commitment first. Unbreakable commitment makes your dreams come true. This isn't only true of weight loss, but other goals as well.

Most people treat their health with a lower priority than their marriage, home, business, or car. They give everything but health a Level Five Commitment. If they do get around to committing to health, they'll give it a Level Two or Three Commitment… maybe.

It is through our bodies that we nurture, experience, and appreciate everyone and everything in life. If we truly care about anything in our lives, then we have to make health a priority. If you've given up having optimal health for a long time, it's hard to realize what you have to lose. If you want sure-fire motivation, you're going to have to think of something else you do have, and put that at risk. If you want to succeed at having the best body you've ever had, it's time to give yourself something to lose.

My Commitment to Your Well-Being

I wrote this book because I'm the kind of guy who lives my life with a sense of purpose and a desire to give service to others. After *Put Your Money Where Your Mouth Is* started working for me, and after I read psychological studies supporting my ideas, I grew determined to share this simple but revolutionary technique with others who have been living with the burden I used to feel.

My new mission is to help end the obesity epidemic. I'm not alone in that mission. There are many players on my team: nutritionists, doctors, researchers, dietitians, nurses, fat farms, diet authors, coaches, and government agencies. I know personally, and have seen in many of my friends, how obesity robs our self-esteem, health, and even life itself. Since I've lost weight, my life has grown in health, freedom, and joy. I don't just feel better in body, but also in mind. I'm accomplishing more in my life today than ever, because I made an unbreakable commitment to losing the weight that was dragging me down physically, emotionally and spiritually. I want to share that transformation with you.

When you diet and fail, the scale goes up and your pride goes down. When you diet and succeed, the scale goes down and your pride goes up. You look good, you feel good, you want to do more, you want to be more, more people are attracted to you, what you have to offer, and life simply becomes more fun. All you need to do to receive those things is to make the most sure-fire commitment of your life. So what are you waiting for?

Chapter 12

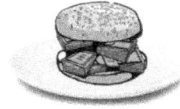

Where Is Your Dinosaur Leading You?

A re you leading your diet, or is your diet leading you? If you've left your reptilian brain in charge, without giving it any motivation beyond its most primitive instincts, then your diet is leading you. Your reptilian brain is terrified of starving, so it will eat like it's starving, even if it's not. If you can give that dinosaur of a brain something else to be afraid of, you can get it to work for you. Then you'll be the one in charge again.

If you keep trying to fight the reptilian brain, you're going to keep losing. The reptilian brain wants to save and hoard all it can. Its job is to survive and reproduce. To the lizard in your head, fat equals energy equals success. Did you know that in ancient Hawaii the king used to be the heaviest man on the island? The reptilian brain is living in an age thousands of years ago. It has not quite caught up with how easy it is to find food—especially the fats and sugars that are necessary to survival, but that in past ages were much harder to come by. Those fats and sugars were never meant to be consumed in the quantities we eat them today, but your lizard brain doesn't know that. All he knows is: "Find, eat, store…Find, eat, store…"

Have you ever consciously watched yourself head to the kitchen when you weren't truly hungry and self-destructively spoon ice cream or peanut butter or chocolate syrup or some other naughty treat into your mouth? Have you ever felt that simultaneous feeling of shame and pleasure, recognizing that you were doing something unhealthy that was going to make your body lumpier and less attractive, while also savoring that creamy, sugary goodness on your tongue? That, my friend, is the reptilian brain in action. That's your inner-dinosaur calling the shots.

The good news is, with the *Put Your Money Where Your Mouth Is* program, you are enlisting the reptilian brain to assist you. You're using your higher order neocortex to create a threat to your survival so big that it will put a scare into your lizard brain. The lizard brain will now trade in its "find, eat, store" survival mode, for an "avoid the threat of disaster" survival mode. When it goes into that mode it will discipline us to avoid eating the crap that it used to obsess about. By creating a commitment that gives you so much to lose, you've given your reptilian brain a new obsession.

The reason this program works is because it recognizes the primitive traits of your brainstem, which have earned such euphemistic names as: reptilian brain, reptilian complex, and primal brain. For better or worse, this part of your brain is responsible for the human instincts and reactions listed below. The neocortex can also play its own role in a few of these areas, but where the reptilian brain is concerned, these processes fall outside our conscious control:

Your Reptilian Brain Is Responsible For:

1. Survival
2. Protection
3. Fight, flight, or freeze response
4. Ritualistic behaviors
5. Tribal associations

6. Resistance to change
7. Involuntary reflexes
8. Power and dominance
9. Territoriality
10. Addictive behavior
11. Status
12. Hunger
13. Shelter
14. Internal body functions
15. Unfiltered eyesight

As you can see, the reptilian complex is not very civilized. It prefers tribalism, rituals, and addictive behaviors. Why do you think you like putting your hand to your mouth so much? Because your inner lizard knows that movement is important to survival. No wonder it's so hard to quit smoking, even with a nicotine patch. That's why you can't just eat one potato chip, even if you're not hungry. The reptilian complex, left to its own devices, is always going to work against your weight loss goals. If you don't rely on a plan that respects this inherent problem, you're never going to succeed at losing weight. Your inner dinosaur doesn't want to lose weight. That's not what he was born to do.

Your Inner Dinosaur Is Not Alone

According to US neuroscientist and physician Dr. Paul McLean, founder of the *Triune Brain Theory*, our brain is actually made up of three kinds of brains. Sometimes these brains have different agendas, and they just don't get along. That's why your diets have failed in the past. When you can get all three components of your brain working together, you will be on your way to success.

When you "think" about whatever you're thinking, that's your neocortex talking, or what some call the rational brain. Sorry to break this to you, but your rational brain is not the most powerful component of who you are. Dr. McLean says the neocortex, also known as the rational brain or mammalian brain, was the last brain to form in the evolution of humankind. Below are some of the thought processes and resulting actions it's responsible for.

Your Rational Brain Is Responsible For:

1. Language
2. Speech
3. Writing
4. Logic
5. Rational thinking
6. Art
7. Sense of Time
8. Planning
9. Voluntary movement
10. Sensory perception

Because the neocortex is the part of the brain that does your thinking, it "thinks" it's in control. Ha ha Ha! Think again. The rational brain only plays a small part in your decision-making process. It has a seat at the table, but doesn't have the biggest say, though it really believes it deserves it. Don't let that thought disillusion you – it doesn't mean you're stupid, or irrational, just that there's a lot more to you than what you think.

Your limbic system also has a seat at the table, but it throws food and cries a lot, because it sits in the emotional seat of the brain. Below are a few things the limbic system is responsible for.

Your Emotional Brain Is Responsible For:

1. Emotions
2. Moods
3. Long-term memory (hippocampus)
4. Emotional association (amygdala)
5. Appetite
6. Sense of smell
7. Bonding needs

Even though emotions are a powerful motivator, even the emotional brain doesn't have as much control over your life as your reptilian brain. The reptilian brain has been around the longest and is responsible for your basic survival, so you can't blame it for having an inflated sense of self-importance. Since it functions without our conscious control, there's not a lot we can do to change its mind once it's made up.

Here's a more representative way to look at your three brains: Imagine a stagecoach in the Old West. The neocortex is the driver holding the reins trying to control the horses the best he can. The brainstem (reptilian brain) is the horses, which have wills of their own and aren't easy to control. The limbic system is the stagecoach, which is peopled with emotions. Some people call that the emotional brain. As long as the driver, the horses, and the cart are all working together and going in the same direction, then the wheels will turn in the right direction and the stagecoach will reach the desired destination.

Your Three Brains:

1. Neocortex - Rational brain
2. Limbic system - Emotional brain
3. Reptilian complex - Primal brain

The *Triune Brain Theory* was first proposed in the 1960's by Dr. Paul McLean. Dr. Carl Sagan boosted its status into pop culture with his 1977 book, *Dragons of Eden*. These very smart people figured out that whenever we make decisions, it requires all three brains to work together. So, although there is one outcome, it represents a community of different needs, perspectives, and languages all vying for position.

When you hear that little voice in your head, that's the rational brain talking. That's the voice that says, "I want to lose 20 pounds." It's also the voice that decides, "If I lower my caloric intake and I workout daily, then I will have success losing 20 pounds." So if your neocortex is so rational, then why have you failed at so many diets? The reason is because the emotional brain and the primal brain were not included in the decision. That's like having one vote out of three and thinking you have a majority.

Much to our rational brain's dismay, the reptilian brain is the one that gets the final say. That's why it's so important to create a high sense of peril when you put a dollar value on your *Put Your Money Where Your Mouth Is* pledges. The reptilian brain responds to danger, so putting yourself at risk of losing big is the best way to get him to vote in favor of following the diet, instead of pulling his own way.

Ultimately, if you want to succeed at weight loss, you need to get all three brains to vote in favor of the same goal. The entire Board of Directors must give your diet unanimous approval. Sometimes, as in real politics, this happens with a little sleight of hand. Each brain has to apply leverage to the other two, based on their motivations and purposes.

So, to figure out the right incentives for these three brains, let's consider what each of them is good at and what each of them wants. The neocortex, or rational brain, can carry on a conversation, plan how to save for college, compute math or science problems, tell jokes, understand time, and can even predict the future to some extent. It even understands the difference between socially appropriate and inappropriate behaviors. Extrapolating from all that, we know that the rational brain can: talk about losing weight, plan a diet to lose weight, compute how many calories in and calories out will lead to weight loss, tell jokes about how hard it is to lose weight, create a deadline for losing weight, and consider how likely it is you'll lose weight based on previous experience. It can even hide embarrassing eating habits.

One thing worth considering is that the rational brain thinks more than 500,000 thoughts per day. If those thoughts are contradictory, it can get confusing in there, even drive a person crazy. That's one reason meditation can be helpful: to keep the brain calm and focused.

The limbic system, or emotional brain, is all about feelings, desires, and urges. It's what makes us feel a fear of public disapproval when we're overweight, happy at the prospect of losing weight, frustrated when we feel limited by a diet, excited when a diet starts to work, sad when we fail to lose weight, or angry at ourselves for not sticking to it. Our emotions can make life both beautiful and terrible, as they give us experiential motivations that move us toward pleasure and away from pain.

The limbic system works together with our reptilian brain to help us survive, as they both try to control the environment we live in to avoid disturbing emotions and pursue pleasant ones. One simple example is the first time you touched a hot stove as a child. Your reptilian brain recognized the pain as contrary to survival and told your reflexes to pull your hand away. Your emotional brain sent you into tears, and planted the experience in your memory so you would remember to keep your hands clear of high heat in the future.

Whatever the three brains think they want, Dr. McLean theorizes that the reptilian brain always casts the deciding vote. If we want all three brains to work together we need to use our rational brain to create a metaphoric hot stove for the emotional brain to fear and the reptilian brain to reflexively avoid. With the *Put Your Money Where Your Mouth Is* plan, our rational brain essentially creates a hot stove that the emotional brain will cue the reptilian brain to avoid. Put another way, this is how we take the reins of the reptilian brain and steer his horses in the direction we want our wagon go.

When we make an agreement in which failure puts us at risk of losing property, pride, social status, or our ability to easily maintain food and shelter, then we ensure our survival-motivated reptilian brain will do its utmost to help us avoid failure. In a diet, our primitive instincts typically work against us, because the reptilian brain still wants to avoid starvation by consuming and storing food whenever possible. By attaching the idea of a diet to all those other things that are contrary to survival, we make our primitive instincts work for us work for us, because the reptilian brain wants to do whatever possible to avoid all those other survival risks.

In tribal times, the threat of losing property, pride, or status could mean losing a desirable mate, which is contrary to the survival instinct of procreation. Those things could also mean losing our place in the tribe. That could lead to a lack of food and shelter, which could mean death, which is also contrary to our survival instincts. Survival is what the reptilian brain is all about. We just have to put something else at risk to convince that old lizard to get on board. You see, if you only put him on a diet, he's just going to worry that you're trying to trick him into starving to death. He wants nothing to do with that: so away run the horses. If he believes that failing to limit his intake of food may lead to even worse consequences, then he'll take you where you want to go.

When you send out that email to three pledge partners promising to lose weight or give up something that costs big bucks, big pride, or big status, you are strapping your reptilian brain into the plan. Your emotions around that promise will keep reminding your reptilian brain to avoid that pain which is contrary to your survival. And your rational brain will be very satisfied with his crafty feat in manipulating those other two jokers: "Well-played, sir!"

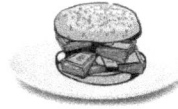

Chapter 13

If At First You Don't Succeed, Up The Ante

If, for some reason, you're not performing well on your diet, then you need to increase the dollar amount or the number of people you have pledged to. It's that simple.

Your emotional brain has decided it wants extra cheese or chocolate or French fries, and your rational brain has allowed a rationalization to slip through to the reptilian brain, revealing that the amount you have to lose in this little wager is survivable. So now your reptilian brain is rebelling. "Aha!" it says. "I knew you were just trying to starve me." And off Mr. Lizard-head goes to stuff you silly with food.

Your reptilian brain always supports you when it's time to make the house payment, the car payment, the insurance payment, and all the rest of the payments that ensure food, shelter, mobility, and the ability to procreate. Your job on this commitment-based diet is to put your weight loss goals on an equal footing with those big-ticket items. If your reptilian friend doesn't see it that way, you just haven't set the price tag high enough. Write those three pledge partners back and tell them you're upping the ante. Take a risk for your health, and go for it!

If the price is high enough, I promise it will work.
If it's not working, you just have not
committed enough.

You need to make your pledge amount as painful to contemplate as if you were a little boy or girl again, being forced to either lose weight or touch that hot stove for a second time—a long, steady, painful second time. That little kid inside you will get the message.

It Ain't Over When It's Over

I learned the importance of making a Maintenance Commitment the hard way. Your pledge to keep the pounds off is just as important as your initial pledge to lose them.

I had reached my goal and neglected to put out a maintenance pledge. That was a big mistake. Without a *Maintenance Commitment*, my reptilian brain chomped at the bit to get back to his old ways. He chomped at the bit until he bit right through it. My inner dinosaur wanted to binge: to eat and drink until he was stuffed. My emotional brain wanted to be merry and free to enjoy whatever the dinosaur indulged in. My rational brain was ready to do the bidding of his two naughty partners by serving up plenty of rationalizations.

**"One drink won't hurt," says the alcoholic.
"One cigarette won't hurt," says the reformed smoker.
"One hand of blackjack won't hurt,"
says the compulsive gambler.**

Alcoholics, smokers, and gamblers have one small advantage in this situation. They can completely abstain from alcohol, tobacco, and games of chance. They'll survive without them. As a former heavy drinker, I know whereof I speak. So what am I saying? I can't survive without popcorn? Of course I can. The problem is that nobody can just quit eating altogether. So the rationalizations come a lot easier.

The reason tomorrow never comes is because tomorrow your reptilian brain will be ready to rope you into a whole new round of rationalizations.

Worse yet, even when we do eat the right things, there's about a 20-minute time delay between the stomach deciding its full and the brain receiving the message. So our bodies are not exactly efficient at telling us when to stop.

Get Mad and Get A Move On

As the numbers on my scale went up, I soon gave up standing on the scale. It's a bad sign when you start avoiding the scale. I told myself everything was fine. It was just a minor setback. I'd get back on track soon. I didn't look that bad. I was lying to myself.

Then I went on a self-destructive rampage.

I had just checked into a hotel in Florida and worked out in the gym. The workout felt great, but I had not eaten much that day and I was starving, so I ordered room service. I decided to have a Caesar salad; you know, the kind that pretends to be healthy vegetables, but is really just an excuse to cram creamy dressing into your mouth? I asked for extra dressing, and sorbet for dessert. Along with that came wonderful bread and, my downfall, butter. I ate all of it, soaking up the extra dressing with the bread. The sorbet was not just a scoop but a whole pint on ice. I guess the room service staff thought I was ordering for two. Feeling disgusted with myself, I sheepishly wheeled the room service table into the hallway and darted back into my room, hoping nobody would see me.

I was embarrassed. I felt like a hypocrite. I had come up with this great weight loss plan and I was planning to share it with the world. That was rock bottom for me, which was a good thing, because it made me mad. Anger isn't always a negative emotion. Anger moves things. In fact, if you've never gotten mad about being fat before, I highly recommend it.

**Get mad about how much you're overeating.
Get mad about how you're out-of-control.
Get so mad that you take action.**

Even though I got mad, I did one other important thing that saved me from plummeting any further. I used my anger to motivate me into action, not to beat myself up. I knew that would send me into a shame spiral, which would send me on another binge. Beating myself up would be beyond counterproductive.

So, what kind of action did I take? I put my rational brain to work on restarting its partnership with my reptilian and emotional brains. I returned to my commitments. I knew that commitment-based dieting worked; I had just failed to set a maintenance pledge. I knew my old habits were right around the corner if I didn't send out my maintenance pledges. Now it was too late to send out a maintenance pledge because I had already put the weight back on. That's the ups and downs of dieting. You get to learn from my mistakes.

So, what kind of action did I take? I called my sons and a couple of other people and I pledged the following:

I will be 177 pounds or less on Valentine's Day 2014. I will also have six-pack abs. If I fail at that goal, I will pay you $1000 plus I run through downtown in my undies.

Thanks for your support. There is nothing you need to do in this agreement except hold me to it.

Sincerely,
I Love You,
Dad

Was it embarrassing for me to write such a letter and push *send*? A little bit.

Did I feel better after writing such a letter and pushing send? Absolutely! I felt inspired. I felt relieved. I knew I was back on track. I knew without a doubt that I was going to have six pack abs. I knew my slender great feeling of health was returning. Wherever your weight loss journey has taken you in the past, let that go. The only place and time any of us can start from is here and now. If you make an unbreakable commitment, right here, right now, and if you're ready to keep remaking that commitment on a maintenance basis, you'll never have to start over again. You'll watch your weight go down, and this time you'll keep it there for good. Congratulations!

Chapter 14

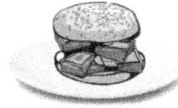

The Success Is Who You Become In The Process

Have you have you ever had a day off and just wasted it? You're at home with no responsibilities, the kids are gone, and you've been planning to use this time to finally get to that cool project that's waiting for you—but you procrastinate. Why not? You have all day. Maybe you lie in bed and read a little, dawdle over a big breakfast, goof around on the Internet, text or call a couple of friends, kick back on the couch to watch a movie or a ballgame, maybe pour yourself a drink and unwind. Before you know it, the sun's going down, and you're a lazy blob who has given up on the day. "Should'ves" and "could'ves" are swirling around in the back of your brain. Then you eat some more or drink some more or watch some more TV until you're comatose and nothing matters.

It can feel so heavenly on the way to hell. Whether we get drunk or high, zone out on TV or the web, or just stuff ourselves with sugar and fat, it feels so good, until it starts to feel bad. By then it's too late. Whatever distractions we choose, sooner or later the consequences catch up with all of us.

I'm offering you a way out of this deadly cycle. The cycle starts with poor planning and lack of accountability. To turn it around, we need a plan; a plan that's set up with deadlines we can't evade, leading to goals we can't afford to fail, tied to standards of accountability that are impossible to ignore.

Even more than personal achievement, I love committing to be part of a goal that's larger than myself and following through. One thing that gets me excited about keeping the weight off is the opportunity to share hope with other people who struggle with food addiction. I want my story to inspire them. Maybe your path to weight loss can be part of a larger story. Maybe you don't want to write a book to motivate others, but maybe losing weight will open the door to coaching your kid's ball team or taking your wife dancing, or inspire you to start a new business or volunteer for a local cause. Mostly, I hope your great feeling of being slender will inspire others to believe that weight loss is actually possible!

Although avoiding pain, danger, and death are important components of survival, so are striving for joy, challenge, and a better life. When we make and keep commitments to improve our lives, it's another way to feed our powerful emotional and reptilian brains. Those two brains really hate to lose, and that's the reason they love to win. The reptilian brain is a survivor, so it loves the idea of competition—which teaches it how to become a better survivor. Our genetic lineage survives better because we overcome obstacles. That's how we learn to win.

Although setting up consequences for failure is crucial to your commitment-based weight loss plan, it's also important to give yourself signposts of success.

I want you to experience the joy of sending off photos of your scale registering the weight you truly want to be. I want you to know the joy of rewarding yourself for success. Dropping a dress-size and having your clothes fit loosely is one of the greatest feelings in the world.

It's true, the possibility of loss is more motivational than the possibility of gain. The opportunity to win is still the second-best motivator for the reptilian brain. Put the two together and it's hard to lose.

Hitch Your Dreams to a Star

Have you ever worried you might get laid off? Have you ever experienced the uncertainty of wondering where your next paycheck was coming from? Have you ever been unemployed? If so, then you know the fear that comes with true uncertainty. Such uncertainty can feed stress, low self-esteem, and the fear of becoming useless. Those are the moments when we fear that we will fall out of favor with our tribe and with the community that values us.

You needn't fear that you will ever become useless to yourself or others, so long as you adhere to one idea: *maintain a sense of purpose.* Your brain wants a purpose, a reason for being, and a challenge to push toward. That's how it's designed to survive and thrive. Once your brain knows it has a purpose of substance and meaning, it will latch onto that for survival. Once others feel the strength of your purpose, they will trust you as a leader, as someone with direction who will always find a way to be useful.

A purpose can be small or big. It can be providing for a family, raising confident children, making people laugh, being of service to clients, repairing machines, helping to solve global warming, striving to feed the homeless, caring for a garden, or just being a good friend. Whatever your purpose, it's important to pave your path with foundational goals that put you in the best position to serve that purpose. Staying physically healthy and fit serves your purpose exponentially.

Weight loss may well be your first step to a greater purpose. What a great incentive to lose weight!

If you're going to accomplish any purpose in life, you have to commit completely to your goals. When it comes to weight loss, the only path to commitment that works is to ensure that you have no option to entertain the alternative. If you have an eating disorder or have failed repeatedly at getting in healthy shape, then you need to make a more unbreakable commitment. If you don't find some way to *Put Your Money* (or whatever is valuable to you) *Where Your Mouth Is*, then you are freewheeling, and that puts you in dangerous territory. If you fly by the seat of your pants, your reptilian brain will take over, and he's not much for long-term planning.

Have you ever thrown a stick for a dog? Remember how happy that dog was when you gave him a simple purpose? "Fetch!" Such a simple goal, yet so fulfilling. The dog was doing something for his master. He was to bring that stick back to you. No matter how hard you threw it again, even into the bushes or water, that faithful dog was ready to sniff around and search every inch of ground until he achieved success. That's how your reptilian brain works. You just have to program it with the purpose you choose.

104

Tell your brain what its purpose is, by writing it down in your pledges. Those pledges tell your brain the quantitative painful loss it will face if it fails. Conversely, knowing the steep price of failure helps your brain recognize the critical importance of success. Once it knows those two things, it will see them as critical to your survival. Your subconscious reptilian brain and limbic system are now on board with what your rational brain wanted all along, and they will do the heavy lifting for you. Together, they will sniff out the diet that works for you. Like a pair of faithful dogs, these powerful aspects of your brain will run together to fetch success and return it to you.

The only way you might fail is if you don't leverage your plan with enough to lose should you fail. If you don't do that, your two subconscious brains won't understand how important this is to you. They won't understand that this is critical to your purpose, and therefore critical to their purpose.

Once I sent out my pledges and declared the highest stakes I could conceive, I gave my inner dinosaur a purpose. He knew where he was going. Once he knew where to go, I knew without a doubt that I was going to hit 177 pounds by Valentine's Day. Once I sent out my pledges, that dinosaur was on board, all the way. Putting it in writing and getting others on board made it inescapable. With that, the dinosaur knew I wasn't kidding. This was serious and this time, I kept him on board for good. I sent out my maintenance pledges with the report of my success!

"The brain is a sugar junkie."
–Jackie Campbell, Heartwood College Nutritionalist

Until I made a Level Five commitment, my desire to lose weight was just a thought blowing in the wind. One of the traits of the reptilian brain is that it has no filter between with it sees and what it perceives. Whenever my dinosaur saw a bear claw in a pastry case, all it saw was the sugar and fat that would feed its immediate survival needs. It didn't see me turning fat or having a heart attack in some fuzzy future that only my high-falutin rational brain could predict or imagine. It only saw what was right in front of it. I had to give more information. Essentially, I had to write down a scary picture and threaten Mr. Dinosaur with that so that he'd know that bear claws are not safe, and that they are a threat to his survival.

On the flip side, he also understood that not eating bear claws would make me, and therefore him, successful. He knew that saying "No" to the scary bear claw would help us survive and thrive, together.

It's a tricky business when the emotional and reptilian brain call on the rational brain to justify their primitive urges. *Sometimes we simply have to outsmart them at their own game.*

Health Alone Won't Motivate Your Dinosaur

We'd all like to feel healthier, look better, and live longer. Those thoughts require putting ideas together that only our rational brain is capable of, and he's not the only one making our decisions. I've put together a list of great reasons to avoid being overweight or obese and to embrace getting healthy and fit. If you read the list, you'll see that it's filled with more than enough reasons to motivate a rational person. Do yourself a favor as you read the list… Ask yourself, "If any rational person would want this, and I have a rational brain, then why have I failed to get in shape?"

These Incentives to Lose Weight Don't Work For the Reptilian Brain:

Looking hot
Increased energy
Moving freely
Enjoying loose-fitting clothes
Long life
Enhanced mood
Self-confidence
Inspiration for greater accomplishments
Glowing skin
Feeling comfortable in your body
Projecting success
Attracting the opposite sex
Better sex
More sex
Better sleep
Fuller participation in life
Increased physical activity
Sense of accomplishment
Fitting into airline seats
Being proud of your body
Receiving compliments
Less aches and pains
Less depression
Better singing
Better whistling

Stronger back and knees
Better blood circulation
More alertness
Less susceptible to sickness and disease
Inspiring others to be healthy
Better employment
More energy
Higher self-esteem
Setting a good example for your children

Everybody wants all these things. So why is it so hard to motivate ourselves to get them? It's because the part of our brain that wants these things is our rational brain, the one that does what we think of as thinking. He's not making our decisions, not alone anyway. Our inner dinosaur and our inner emotional child are in on this too, and neither of them are deep thinkers. Oh sure, the emotional brain will get excited about some of these things, until something shiny distracts him: like butter, or a greasy burger, or soda. You can try talking sense into that big baby and that dinosaur. It won't do much good. Terms like health, longevity, and obesity mean nothing to them. They don't ponder the mysteries of the future. The dinosaur can't imagine a body that looks and feels different from the one you have now; and the baby can't understand delayed gratification.

Ultimately, your inner dinosaur is in charge, and all he understands are things like: eat = live, starve = die; warm = live, freeze = die; tribe = live, alone = die. So you have appeal to that side of him.

Modern psychology is very clear on what it takes to do that. Pain and loss are stronger motivators than gain and accomplishment. If it hurts too much our dinosaur won't do it. That's how he fights for basic survival. He's wired to stay away from pain.

Neal Cole, a leader in the field of market research has learned a lot about loss aversion during his more than twenty years of experience. He has discovered that human beings are intrinsically afraid of loss, to the point that they hate losing much more than they love winning. So, when humans make choices, the fear of loss will loom larger than the hope of success in their decision-making process. He has found this to be true even when the monetary value of what someone has to lose is identical to what they have to gain. If the opportunity arises to play a game in which you stand to win $100 or lose $100, most people won't play.

If an option poses a potential loss that could be ruinous or threaten their lifestyle, people will normally dismiss the option completely.

In the case of the *Put Your Money Where Your Mouth Is* diet system, your rational brain is able to use this fear in your favor. It understands that there's something larger at stake, so it makes the promise before the reptilian brain knows what's happening. The rational brain creates a major loss as a consequence for failure, so the reptilian brain has no choice but to win. If it had a choice, it wouldn't play at all. Your rational brain is the one that pushed the send button, and the reptilian brain is stuck playing along. The promise is made, and the reptilian brain can't take it back. Too many other survival needs are at stake. It has to keep its word. It has to maintain its ties to the tribe.

Why Make Such a Scary Wager?

Your body is your home. It's where you live 24 hours a day. When your house is a mess, it's difficult to be happy. When your house is tidy, in good repair, and well furnished, then life rocks.

When I walk around old neighborhoods, I find it interesting to think about what sets apart the homes that are in beautiful shape and the homes that are run down. We forget sometimes, living in the moment, that all of the houses looked spiffy when they were built first. The ones that are run-down didn't get that way in just a few months, or even in just a few years. It happened slowly over a long period of time. It may have happened so slowly that the owner failed to notice how dilapidated his or her house was becoming.

Maybe you just woke up to how far your body has fallen into disrepair, or maybe you've known for a long time. You'd probably be hard-pressed to remember the moment it all started, or the moment when it became so hard to turn back. Maybe you're body isn't that far gone. Maybe you just need to shed another twenty-five pounds. Yet something that simple can be difficult. Why?

In my real estate business one of my specialties was fixer-uppers. I would buy a run-down house for an extra-low price, put in a small injection of cash and some "sweat equity" to modernize the building, and then sell it for a profit. Has your body become a fixer-upper? The good news is that if all you need to do is lose weight, then it can be fixed. The bad news is that nobody else can make the decision to fix it but you. It has to be you. You have to make a level five commitment. If you've been stuck sitting on the couch or standing at the refrigerator for a long time, then fixing your fixer-upper is going to call for you to overcome inertia.

"An object at rest tends to stay at rest..."
– Sir Isaac Newton
"A blob on the couch tends to stay on the couch."
– Daniel Miller

The idea of the *Put Your Money Where Your Mouth Is* pledges is to create a powerful crowbar to overcome your inertia, to pry you off that couch, to push you away from that fridge. All three of your brains—rational, emotional, and reptilian— may well wonder why they should put such a large stash of cash at risk to make that happen. They're risk averse. You have to give your rational brain sway only long enough to understand that once it sets the promise in motion, the other two brains will ensure that it doesn't lose. You only have to remind your rational brain that if you don't take the risk, your entire quality of life, and perhaps your life itself is at stake.

---

*You only need convince yourself of that fact
just long enough to write that pledge
and send it to three people.*

Once you set those pledges in motion, they'll set your body in motion. Another thing good old Sir Isaac taught us is that once a body is in motion, it tends to stay in motion.

Your body is not only your home, it's your mode of transportation. It gets you around on the planet. When you have a great car, it's so much fun to go places. When your car is old and beat up, sometimes it breaks down before it gets there. What kind of a day do you have when your car won't start?

The way you care for your actual home and car says a lot about you. You can't hide them. The same goes for the home and vehicle that is your body. Yet many Americans spend their health to afford a beautiful home and car, than spend their wealth trying to get back their health.

Your pledge is not just a pledge to lose weight.
It's a pledge to realign your priorities.

Imagine yourself in that slender body of your dreams right now. Hear the conversations about the changes you've made going on around you. Feel the looseness of your clothes and the vibrancy of your energy within. See yourself dancing lightly in your kitchen in the joy of who you have become in accomplishing this dream. Stay with this image and bring it back on a daily basis as you make this journey to the new you that you are about to become. Congratulations on your success!

Chapter 15

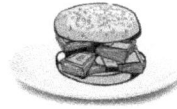

Creating The Pressure
That Pushes You

I recently attended a marketing convention where many wealthy people were in attendance. An alarming number of them were overweight. Why is it that people work on their wealth more than they work on their health? However much money they make, it will be meaningless to them when they're dead.

On the other hand, I did notice that the most successful people in the room tended to be trim and fit. Maybe those who are most committed to success understand that it's a complete package: that you can't succeed *in* life unless you succeed *at* life. I think it's even simpler than that.

Highly successful people have learned to train their brains by making commitments that carry big stakes. Sure, making money and having power are great incentives, but when they play in the big leagues they live with the constant threat of big losses and public failure. They're experts at Level Five Commitments: public commitments, in writing, with big money and personal reputations on the line.

The Threat of Death Isn't Enough

What is the immediate pain or threat of overeating? Not much, besides heartburn. Over time, becoming overweight can be very painful: making us uncomfortable in our clothes, embarrassed in front of people, exhausted from carrying around excess weight, unable to join in fun activities. Over time, becoming obese can be life-threatening, leading to such health problems as diabetes, heart attack and stroke. However the key word here is "time." Most of the pain and health risk associated with obesity arrives very slowly over a long period of time. We grow accustomed to the pain because the pain grows slowly upon us.

If I woke up one morning 30 pounds heavier than I was the day before, I would freak out. I would definitely do something about it—right now! I'd go see my doctor. "Do you think it's a tumor, Doc? Something terrible is wrong!"

Instead we suffer losses gradually. Our rational brain understands that any number of the bad things listed below might be on the way, but our primitive reptilian brain just isn't enough of a long-term planner to care. He doesn't even understand time.

These Down-the-road Threats Don't Motivate Weight Loss in the Reptilian Brain:

1. Heart attack
2. Diabetes
3. High blood pressure
4. Stroke
5. Sleep apnea
6. Snoring
7. Clogged arteries
8. Colon cancer
9. Breast cancer
10. Osteoarthritis

11. Hyperventilation syndrome
12. Reproductive problems
13. Gallstones
14. Back pain
15. Knee pain
16. Shortness of breath
17. Not getting "checked out" by the opposite sex
18. Giving up an active lifestyle
19. Playing catch with your kids
20. Fitting into your cool clothes
21. Leaving your family to buy an oversized coffin

Some of the above problems are enough to motivate people to lose weight, but often that's only *after* they happen. Until then, overweight or obese people tend to trudge along in mild pain and shame. I recently talked to a man who lost 200 pounds. Why? Because he had a heart attack. Surely he knew before that happened that being 200 pounds overweight would put him at a greater risk of a heart attack. So why didn't he choose to lose the 200 pounds *before* it happened?

I believe that his primal brain just didn't have the imagination to picture that potentially fatal moment in his future. It wasn't until he actually experienced the pain in his heart and had the opportunity to peer over the cliff of impending death that he felt motivated to change. The benefits of being healthy had never motivated him enough to change. It had taken fear and pain to do that. Fear is more motivating than hope. Pain is more motivating than pleasure. Overweight people get so used to their discomfort, that it starts to seem comfortable to them. So they stay there until something scares them out of that "comfort zone." Humans have a high tolerance for pain, which is good for survival, except when it comes to losing weight.

If we want to motivate ourselves to leave an uncomfortable situation to which we've become accustomed, we need to create an artificial pain that is bigger than the pleasure of the yummy sugary or fatty treats that are so readily available to most of us. That's the idea behind *Put Your Money Where Your Mouth Is*.

To Motivate Yourself: Increase Pain, Not Gain

Tony Robbins says that emotions make up the quality of our lives. The emotions associated with being fit and trim are wonderful. It's easier to feel self-confident, optimistic, and joyful when it's easy to get out of bed in the morning, enjoy a brisk walk or bike ride during the day, and go dancing or have great sex at night. Emotions tend to slide into low self-esteem, pessimism, and depression when it's hard to simply unroll from the seat of a car. Why do we put up with such negative emotions?

Think of a time when you did something that you were ashamed of. Did you want to run away and hide? That's basically what addicts do: alcoholics hide in booze, drug addicts hide in drugs, and over-eaters hide in food. Some people do all three. They can only hide so long before they have to come up for air. The real world and their real feelings are always still there, waiting for them.

This becomes a vicious cycle: becoming drunk, high, or overweight leads to shame over our behavior or appearance, which leads us to hide in more booze, drugs, or food, which leads to more shame, and so on. The addict's health goes down-hill. The couch springs grow weak from overuse. The blood slows. This all happens in tiny increments over time. Unless something intervenes, decreasing health is inevitable.

Ask anyone in advertising and they'll tell you that the fear of pain is stronger than the hope of gain. That's why so many commercials make us feel inadequate for not having what all the smart, pretty, successful people seem to have. That's why our reptilian brain would rather sit home and stay fat than walk into the gym and face the humiliation of being seen. Sure we might not get to be smart, pretty, and successful: but we're used to that, and now we're just invested in making sure nobody finds out.

That is why it is so important to leverage the priorities of the reptilian brain by heaping on the threat of immediate pain, should we fail at achieving the body we actually want. That's why we need to make the "ouch" of staying overweight inevitable and excruciating. We need to create commitments with consequences for failure that are completely unacceptable to the reptilian brain.

If we truly want to lose weight and keep it off, we have to set ourselves up so that failure is not an option.

Past Failures Don't Matter

I don't care how many times you've gained and lost weight, and neither should you. When it comes to your commitment to losing weight, the only thing that matters is what you do right now. You will not make your commitment any stronger by beating yourself up over the past. Your commitment must be about the near future. Everything in your past is now just the learning experience that brought you to this moment.

If you were a success at everything you did in life, your life would be a boring, flat line of sameness. If everything you ever did were gauged a success, it would lose its luster; and then who would bother with success? Losing weight is not easy, nor should you want it to be. If you want to achieve something, then why bother unless you're achieving something special? If this were easy there would be no fat people.

We all know that life is a journey, but don't forget that your body is the vehicle that takes you on this journey. Take care of that vehicle and keep it in top shape, and it will take you to amazing places, making your journey on this planet a joyous adventure. Fail to take care of it, and you not only limit the places you can go, but run the risk of ending up broken down on the side of the road, going nowhere. Maybe knowing that hasn't helped you change your habits in the past. All you need is to let it motivate you for the few minutes it will take to write and send your pledges. At that point, your primal brain's fear of pain and loss will kick in and keep you on track.

If you are overweight, then your life is not as good as it could be. Your first step to change is to love yourself for exactly who you are right now. From that point on, make your pledges to lose weight or else, and send them. Now is the only place you can start from, so don't let what has gone before convince you that you can't do this. If you start this from a place of self-loathing, you're not going to have the courage to send those pledges. Start with self-acceptance. Know that you're at the perfect place to start.

Scare Yourself Skinny

What is the missing link between you now and you 20, 40, or 100 pounds lighter? It is all possible. It's not willpower. It's commitment.

Do you think you would run faster to escape an attacking lion or to get to Disneyland? Would you run faster to save your child from a tornado or to reach a sale at Macy's? Would you run faster to escape an IRS audit or to get to a bank that offers 7% interest? You will run much faster from the thing you *fear* than you will toward the thing you want. Your *Put Your Money Where Your Mouth Is* pledge is leveraging that fear factor. You are going to scare yourself skinny by threatening yourself with a major loss. That loss is going to motivate you to run from those cravings—at least more often than not.

Your* Put Your Money Where Your Mouth Is *pledges are commitments that keep you on track by leveraging that most powerful tool of human nature: fear.

All you need to do is step out of your comfort zone for three minutes, the length of time it takes to write your pledges and send them to three people. Do it now.

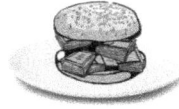

Chapter 16

How Much Weight? Who To Pledge, How Much Money? How Much Time?

Your unbreakable commitment only requires four decisions from you: 1) how much weight you want to lose, 2) by when, 3) how much you need to wager on your success to make yourself too scared to fail, and 4) which three people to send your pledges to. Once you make those decisions, write those pledges, and send them. Then you are off and running.

I suggest losing 1/2 pound to 1 pound a week. That's a realistic and healthy goal. I also suggest you factor an extra two or three weeks into your deadline to give you time to shop around to find a weight loss program you like.

There's a huge world of diets out there, and all sorts of toys, tools, and support systems to go with them. It can get extremely confusing. I suggest you keep it simple: pick one and follow it exactly. Although you will probably cheat, that's why you have your pledges. Use your pledges to help you stay on track and keep you from getting distracted long term. If you fall off the horse, just get right back on—but then, once you send the pledges you won't need me to convince you to do that, your fear of losing will convince you.

Who to pledge: Pledge anyone who is important to you. Pledge anyone who is not important to you. Pledge anyone you know. I've found it doesn't really matter who you pledge. I've pledged my kids and friends who live in different states. I've pledged my next door neighbor. You can always pledge me… it just doesn't matter. What's important is that you send out your pledges ASAP.

How Much money should I pledge? Pledge a little more than you can afford to lose. Be outrageous. Pledge a crazy embarrassing action on top of your monetary pledge. Be creative. When you come up with your own unique pledging idea, please do me a favor and email it to me so I can include it in the web site or the next edition of this book.

Here are some examples of inventive, cherished items you might pledge in a Level Five Commitment:

1. Family heirlooms
2. Find silverware and china
3. Nice furniture
4. Your bed
5. Your pets
6. Your watch
7. Your iPhone
8. Your truck
9. Any prize possessions you have that other people like

How much time should I give myself? I like to break it up into little bites. Go for losing 10 to 25 pounds at a time. Baby steps. When you send out your success photos, simply pledge the next baby step of your weight loss program to the same 3 people. This will build your confidence and self-esteem. For example, if your overall goal is to lose 60 pounds, then break that up into 3 sections of 20 pounds each. This will give you 3 celebrations and 3 wins. Don't forget to send out the 6 month maintenance pledge when you hit your final goal weight.

There are just a few thousand of ways of losing weight and getting in shape that I'm familiar with. I've found that my greatest key to success has been surrounding myself with a community and not trying to do it all by myself. If you're shy about this, don't worry. It doesn't take much to make that first step into joining a group. Just joining a gym or fitness center can help you step into the momentum of working out with other people. Even if you don't know who they are, you are in a roomful of people who are all focused on a similar goal: getting in shape. That positive, communal vibe can be very affirming during the difficult, sometimes lonely process of losing weight.

When you're first getting in shape, you may not feel you have the motivation, self-confidence, or knowledge to walk into a gym and start a workout routine. That's one reason I believe that exercise classes and personal trainers offer wonderful support systems.

Don't underestimate how much easier it is to get in shape if you pick activities and exercises that are fun for you. For example, maybe you hate jogging or going to the gym, but maybe you like hiking and dancing. If so, then hike up mountains and dance, dance, dance. Remember, if you're going to change your body, you have to throw yourself into this. So, if you're only dancing or hiking once a week, you'll need to find additional intense activities to keep you firing on all cylinders.

The jury is out on how helpful supplements are in general. I believe it depends on the supplement. If you want to try them, talk to your doctor. Personally, I find several supplements helpful. The body is a chemical stew, and some of the supplements I use are effective at "tricking" the body into shedding fat cells faster. Others simply help keep the body's operating at peak health and efficiency to alleviate the tired feeling that we can sometimes encounter when losing weight.

Whatever approach you choose to help you get through this diet, remember it has to be something you can stick with—because you're the one who made this commitment and you're the one who is responsible for getting yourself through this. If you find strength in prayer then pray. If meditation helps you focus, then meditate. If affirmations enhance your confidence, then write down affirmations on sticky notes and scatter them all over the house. Whatever you do, I highly recommend writing down your goals, both long-term and short term every day. When you write them down, it helps you to see them as realities and it helps you to stay focused. Whatever, you do, pull out all the stops. Remember, failure is not an option, so whatever it takes to succeed: do it.

Some diet programs tell you exactly what to eat, or ship prepackaged food to you. If you have major issues with self-control, then maybe this is a good approach for you. Other diet programs simply give you calorie targets, or food groups to prioritize. That can be good for people who freak out when they feel deprived. Meanwhile, other programs leverage our desire to be part of a like-minded group. I went to the holistic health Institute in San Diego and did a wheatgrass cleanse with about 100 people. It was tough at first; but it felt transformational by the end.

Meanwhile, if you need total support and can afford it, there are institutions that allow you to check in and completely retreat from the temptations and distractions of the world. Just remember, you'll have to figure out how to commit to keeping the weight off when you return to the regular world. Whatever approach you choose, remember that this won't work long term unless you change your habits long term. Once you've lost the weight, sending out your weight maintenance pledges is critical.

Whatever diet you choose, whatever exercise you use, remember to smile smile smile smile smile. *Your attitude is going to help you get through this*, and when you smile, you give your body a signal that what you are doing for it is good, not bad. Love yourself for what you're doing. Celebrate every little win. That joy is going to help push you toward success, and away from failure. Fear may make a more surefire motivator, but joy is ultimately what makes this worth your while.

Momentum is the Magic Word

New doors of success begin to open to you after make your commitment. It doesn't happen by itself. Starting a diet, signing up for a martial arts class, joining a support group: These sorts of things are what help you to build momentum to move away from failure and toward your goal

It's tough to break bad habits. That's why you need to lean on your commitments, to help you push through that initial resistance. I promise when you get to the other side of the resistance you'll begin to discover a powerful side of yourself. It's the part of yourself that knows you are worthy and amazing. Don't expect it to happen overnight. Go slow. Going fast is like giving yourself permission to self-destruct from pressure. Whatever you do, don't hurt yourself! You might think that pushing yourself hard will give you faster or better results. It also increases the risk of injury, which will ultimately make this whole process harder.

Remember you've committed to losing this weight. Injury will not get you out of the commitment. There is no clause for injury in your pledges, or at least, there shouldn't be. That would make it too easy for your subconscious to try to trip you up and get you out of doing the hard work.

I do have a self-destructive side, and since you're reading this book, I'm guessing you have one too. Why pretend it isn't there? That hasn't helped you in the past. If you want to succeed, you need to be aware of the ways in which you're capable of getting in your own way. Beware of that side of you that wants to pretend it's in control, that wants to say, "I've got this handled, no problem, I can take care of this myself!" as an excuse for giving in to an old habit.

You will cheat. It's inevitable. Don't use that as an excuse to give up. If you made your pledges big enough, then you can't afford to. When you fall off that horse, get right back on. If you find you're not getting back on the horse, then I'm sorry but you haven't put a big enough dollar amount on your pledges. So send out some new ones. Create some more leverage for yourself. Do whatever it takes to pressure yourself to follow through.

Whatever you do, get out of your comfort zone! Life does not happen in the comfort zone. Do new things every day. Push yourself just a little harder every day. Don't go over the edge. Just a little push. Do it every day. Push through the resistance until you start to feel the momentum. That momentum will build on itself and make the journey easier. Momentum will make the journey more fun. Momentum is your friend.

If your life is a journey, then change is an adventure. You can make dieting a painful punishment or a daring adventure. It's up to you. You can choose to cry at your mistakes or laugh at yourself. I say, laugh! Don't take yourself too seriously. If you're the heaviest person in the gym, big deal! Somebody else at that gym was once in your shoes. Just smile and keep on walking, riding, running, sweating, stretching, swinging, and dancing. Find some little teeny tiny way to enjoy the process, and then find another one.

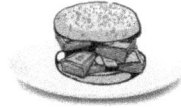

Chapter 17

Leveraging Your Money And Your Tribe

Since I first began creating the *Put Your Money Where Your Mouth Is* program, many studies have confirmed that betting on yourself is a powerful tool for personal change. Researchers have discovered that people have greater success at weight loss when something else besides their health is at stake—when they have something tangible to lose if they fail.

Part of the reason this sort of wager works is because it increases the stakes, so that our primal brains become more invested in avoiding food. Another reason it works is because it requires involving other people in our commitment. To make a Level Five Commitment requires reaching outside of the gray matter between your ears and inviting somebody else to be part of your process. Humans are tribal. We thrive in community. Humans find it easier to complete tasks when they work together.

Folks, this is only the beginning. Try it out for yourself. Be bold. You don't need to be part of a big study. You don't need to be part of a university. All you need to do is send out three emails to three people telling them that you will be a certain weight by certain date or you will pay them a certain amount of cash. It's as simple as that. Scientists are just starting to understand why it works. One thing they now know is that it does work.

Your Wager Creates a Support Group

When you send out your Level Five Pledges to three people, it is not just the fear of losing money that provides your incentive to lose weight. Your other incentive comes from your new tribe. That's right, when you send out those pledges, you are initiating at least three people, plus your mutual friends, into your tribe. You might think that tribe would be rooting against you. After all, they stand to make a tidy profit if you fail. I've found that's not what happens. Your pledges motivate your pledge partners to root for you.

After I sent out my pledges, sometimes I got together with my pledge partners, and yes they did tease me, coaxing me to go off my diet: "Hey Daniel, have some cheesecake!" "Hey, Daniel, try my artichoke dip! It's really good. I made it myself." So it sounds like people trying to lure me to failure, right? Wrong. Even though these friends each stood to gain $1000 if I did not meet my weight goals, it was clear that they were teasing me as a playful way to show me they knew I could do it. It was all in good fun. It was an opportunity to laugh together. It was a ritual game that told me we were all in on the joke together and they were on my side. I had strengthened my support by creating a new tribe.

All that joking temptation from people who stood to gain if I failed actually made me feel more supported than if I had just kept my diet goals a secret. I had created a support group. My pledge letters became more like recruitment letters, creating a team that wanted me to win.

The scientific evidence is building. Making a wager that leverages your fears and your friendships is a powerful tool in weight loss. Use the science. Use it for weight loss. Use it to quit

130

smoking. Use it to quit drugs. Use it to curb any bad habit in your life.

We're just beginning to understand the mysteries of the human brain. We're just beginning to understand how the chemicals in our body work. We're just beginning to understand how to use this science to attain good health. For now, we only know that it works, and that it's good for your health. If that's not enough to convince you, I don't know what is.

Blessings On Your Journey

As my grandpa always said, "Your health is your wealth." There's nothing better than feeling good, unless it's to help others feel good too. If you're not healthy, then it's very difficult to serve mankind. It's through service that we really find our joy. I hope this book is of service to you.

We only get so many days on this planet. Most of us can likely increase that number by decreasing our weight and increasing our health. When our bodies are healthier, we can certainly enjoy our days more.

May the joys that you used to find through overindulging in food and drink transform into joys of indulging in walks, runs, dance, yoga, and other forms of healthy, creative activity. May the highs that come with having a great body become the fireworks that celebrate your life. May you attract the knowledge, tools, and support you need to follow through on this new commitment. May you stay inspired throughout the process. May you grow in spirit. May the mysterious wonders of the universe bless you on your journey.

Acknowledgements

Special thanks goes out to all those who helped make this dream come true: Mark, Cara, Anne, Jim, Rob, Dad, Erykah, Micheal, Nate, Rylie, Kathleen, Uncle Micheal, Mom, Tom, Katie, Justina, Harry, Jake, Marshal, Ian, Lianne, Jennifer, Stephanie, Jimmy, My Heartwood Family, My Amazing Community, Chad, JT, Wayne, Matt, John, Liana, and Lorrie.

About the Author

Daniel R. Miller was born during a blizzard in Omaha, Nebraska while his family was passing through town on their way home to California. Their departure was further delayed due to Daniel contracting pneumonia in the process. His hospital visit was extended for several months, and he had to be incubated, living in a "bubble." Throughout his life his family often joked they were "not sure what happened in that bubble," but it was only the beginning of a unique path of growth, personal development, discovery, and transformation.

Daniel's family eventually moved to Phoenix, Arizona where he spent most of his childhood. Daniel excelled in sports, acting, and television there. Daniel attended the University of Arizona. He studied Art and Business. Daniel furthered his education at the Heartwood College of Northern California. He majored in Transformational Therapies and earned specialized certifications in Nutrition, Polarity Therapy, and Hypnotic Counseling.

Daniel met his wife at school at Heartwood. They traveled and studied extensively in India and Nepal. Then later venturing to Olympia, Washington, where they had two sons, Nate, and Rylie. They established the revered "Burrito Heaven" and the accompanying "Tequila Bar" teaching the native Olympians the art of Tequila-ology.

Moving back to Northern California, the Millers created businesses around forest restoration, tree planting, and real estate. Always educating himself along the way, Daniel studied with Tony Robins, Marshal Silver, Jerry and Ester Hicks, T Harv Ecker, and Landmark Education.

Daniel is an avid coach, having worked through over nine seasons of baseball, football, and basketball. He developed wooden "build from scratch" learning toys for preschool children. He regularly participates in community services. One of his proudest achievements was helping build a community theater dedicated to a group of individuals in his home town.

Daniel's believes "Service is where the growth is; it is out of our struggles that we grow and learn the most." He sincerely hopes his past education and life experience can be a match to your needs in this ever changing world.

www.ingramcontent.com/pod-product-compliance
Lightning Source LLC
Chambersburg PA
CBHW022114280326
41933CB00007B/388